CANDIDA ALBICANS
Could Yeast Be Your Problem?

Shows how the proliferation of the yeast *Candida* in the body
has been found to be the root of illness when no obvious cause
is evident.

DATE DUE

CANDIDA ALBICANS
Could Yeast Be Your Problem?

Leon Chaitow, D.O., N.D.

Healing Arts Press
One Park Street
Rochester, Vermont 05767

Healing Arts Press
One Park Street
Rochester, Vermont 05767

Copyright © 1985, 1987, 1988 by Leon Chaitow

LIBRARY OF CONGRESS CATALOGING IN PUBLICATION DATA

Chaitow, Leon,
    Candida albicans : could yeast be your problem? / by Leon Chaitow.
       p.   cm.
    Bibliography: p.
    Includes index.
    ISBN 0-89281-247-8 (pbk.)
    1. Candidiasis—Popular works.   2. Candida albicans—Popular
works.   I. Title.
    RC123.C3C48   1988
    616.9'69—dc19   88-23540
                                                                    CIP

                Printed and bound in the United States
                     20   19   18   17   16   15

Healing Arts Press is a division of Inner Traditions International, Ltd.

Distributed to the book trade in the United States by Harper and
                        Row Publishers, Inc.

Distributed to the book trade in Canada by Book Center, Inc.,
                        Montreal, Quebec

Distributed to the health food trade in Canada by Alive Book,
                     Toronto and Vancouver

ACKNOWLEDGMENTS

The pioneering research of Dr. C. Orion Truss in the uncovering of Candida's involvement in a wide range of diseases and conditions deserves recognition. I respectfully dedicate this book to him. Others who have made major contributions to our knowledge about Candida, and to whom I owe a debt, include Dr. William G. Crook and Dr. Jeffrey Bland. I have quoted from the works of all three of these respected scientists, and thank them on behalf of all those who will benefit from their original research. The books of Dr. Truss and Dr. Crook (*The Missing Diagnosis* and *The Yeast Connection*, respectively) are particularly worthy of study by anyone who wishes to have a deeper understanding of this subject.

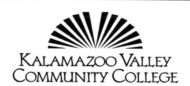

CONTENTS

1

Candida Yeast and
Common Health Problems

Recently, it has become clear that a great many common health problems, both physical and mental, might have a common cause—namely, the spread in the body of a yeast that lives in each and every one of us. Its name is *Candida albicans*; and we will call it Candida for short.

Because it is present in all people from about the age of six months, doctors tend to overlook Candida as the cause of various diseases or conditions. Because it occurs in everyone, it would seem that Candida could not cause health problems in only some. This reasoning has diverted attention from Candida, except in rare conditions in which it proliferates to such an extent as to become life-threatening. This critical condition often happens in people whose immune system has been weakened by disease or drugs (in therapy or in abuse). However, many people may indeed be suffering from a less-pronounced spread of Candida, which, while not sufficient to endanger life, is certainly enough to produce a wide array of debilitating symptoms. These include depression; anxiety; unnatural irritability; digestive symptoms such as diarrhea, constipation, bloating, and heartburn; tiredness and a sense of hopelessness; allergies; acne; migraine; cystitis; vaginitis; thrush; and menstrual problems and premenstrual tension.

The key to understanding the way in which this vast array of symptoms could possibly be caused by a yeast that lives in all of us lies in an appreciation of the factors that can encourage a spread of yeast. In most people there is an uneasy truce between their bodies and the yeast. For most of us an equilibrium exists. The yeast can live—even thrive—and present no problems to its host, as long as it is confined to specific sites. Should it go beyond these sites, the defense capability of the body, as represented by its immune system in general and its white blood cells in particular, attacks and destroys the yeast. There are also actual physical barriers, such as the mucous lining of the digestive tract, which prevents intrusion through it by yeast or any other undesirable elements. All mucous membranes contain further protective substances that can destroy invading particles of yeast. We will consider these defenses later, in our search for an understanding of Candida.

Health problems arise when, because of one of a variety of causes, the body's defense capability becomes deficient or weakens. Should this happen, the controls that keep Candida in check are removed, and the yeast can spread to areas that are normally out of bounds. If at the same time the foods the yeast thrives on happen to be in plentiful supply, we have the right environment for an explosion of Candida activity. This is precisely the combination of factors that has become widespread in Western society over the past twenty-five to thirty years. The introduction of broad-spectrum antibiotics, the use of the contraceptive pill, and the widespread use of steroids, have all played their part in Candida's growth. In addition the increase in the use of sugar and sugar-rich foods has provided the yeast with just the sustenance it needs. This unfortunate combination of factors is the root cause of yeast-related symptoms for many people.

To understand Candida, a careful look at the nature of the enemy is necessary, together with consideration of those factors and circumstances that allow it to proliferate, and what the consequences of such a proliferation might be. We will look at the dietary aspect of Candida in detail, and also at those changes in medical care that have inadvertently allowed Candida's new-found freedom from adequate surveillance and control. We will then be in a position to consider methods of controlling Candida. Fortunately this is the brighter side of the sorry mess. Because it seems unlikely that the causative elements of the picture are going to be removed from the population at large, the fact that control is possible, in the majority of cases, is a blessing indeed.

It should be clearly understood that I am not suggesting that the conditions I have listed are always the result of Candida infection. It is certainly true that all of them *might* be such a result, but they can have other causes. The view of those practitioners now aware of the possibility of Candida's involvement in common disease problems of this sort is that when a combination of such symptoms appears with no other obvious causes apparent, Candida should be the prime suspect. Unlike most infections and infestations, it is not really possible to test for the presence of Candida to prove or disprove such an assumption. This is because, as has already been stated, Candida is present to some extent in all of us. Thus, looking for it is as pointless as looking for mice in a granary; they are always present, but in what number? Candida is so ubiquitous that microbiologists ususally ignore it when they come across it. The way to prove that a condition (or a cluster of conditions) is the result of Candida is to treat it, and if the symptoms disappear, the proof is irrefutable.

Here is one of the very few instances in which the treatment is the main means of diagnosis. The initial suspicions that result in the treatment rely upon recognizing the symptoms that the presence of Candida might produce, as well as an awareness of those factors that influence Candida's development and behavior. This knowledge, combined with a thorough history of previous and current medical treatment and drug usage, as well as diet and stress factors, will give clear indications as to the likelihood, or otherwise, of Candida being a possible culprit.

We are going to explore these areas in order to formulate a series of recommendations for the control of Candida and for the prevention of its accompanying complications.

The exaggeration of a previously fairly harmless interaction between ourselves and a yeast is one of the complications of civilization, and as such is rapidly becoming so widespread as to constitute an epidemic. The failure, thus far, by all but a handful of doctors to recognize the situation is tragic, for the degree of human suffering involved is enormous. Prevention is not difficult, and control, while a slow process, is not beyond the limits of any intelligent individual.

The major credit for unraveling the mystery of Candida belongs to one man, who recognized that what he was seeing in his own patients had worldwide importance. First he diligently assembled his evidence, which he presented in a scientific journal (the *Journal of Orthomolecular Psychiatry*). He then returned to his investigation. Over a period of years, his results, involving an enormous range of diseases, from acne to schizophrenia to what appeared to be multiple sclerosis, were so impressive that the world beat a path to his door. Dr. C. Orion Truss, of Birmingham, Alabama, will be remembered for his work in this field by tens of thousands of grateful people. His masterly investigation and research, conducted in a typical medical practice, shows how important simple observation is in the quest for knowledge and the understanding of Man's ills. Truss has written his own story of his search, and the whole story of Candida, in his book *The Missing Diagnosis*. That book and an excellent book on the same subject by another renowned practitioner, Dr. William Crook, entitled *The Yeast Connection*, both recommend the use of an antifungal drug called nystatin for controlling yeast. They also suggest other methods, including nutrition and desensitization.

This book, however, does not suggest the use of drugs, but instead presents alternatives to the use of nystatin. This is not to say that nystatin should never be used, only that in most cases there are ways of restoring the body's ability to fight the yeast. There are also naturally occurring nutrients that further help to control the wildly proliferating yeast. Hence the reason for this book, for in every other way the two books mentioned above are excellent, and are valuable contributions to the literature on health.

Our task here is to observe the nature of the enemy, what makes it active, and how to recognize its activity. Only then will we be able to learn how to deal with it.

2

Candida and Your Defense System

The object of our interest is a member of the yeast family. Strictly speaking, it is a member of a subgroup of the family of plants known as fungi or molds. Yeasts live practically everywhere on our planet, deriving their nutrients from most organic sources. This means anything that is alive, or has been alive, can support yeasts. Rather than having roots like other plants, yeasts derive their nutrients via the use of enzymes. Given the right conditions for growth and replication, yeast is capable of almost explosive growth, as anyone who has made bread will testify.

Roger Williams,[1] a world-renowned research scientist, states that if a single yeast cell were given a highly favorable environment, with a good assortment of nutrients and the correct temperature, it could, within twenty-four hours, produce a colony of over a hundred yeast cells. At this rate of reproduction, Williams calculates that within one week, one cell could turn into a yeast colony weighing one billion tons. The fact that this does not happen, and is not likely to happen, is because the environment is seldom ideal for any creature on earth, least of all for yeast. The rapid growth rate does, however, highlight a point pertinent to our understanding of Candida. It seldom takes over the entire body, but when it does, the consequences are serious. Candida can spread only if the environment for it is excellent, and if the body's defense mechanisms are weakened or absent.

Williams points out that in nature, yeast cells are almost always hampered by imperfect or inadequate environmental conditions. Otherwise, they would have engulfed the earth long ago. The same factors control the colonies of Candida (and other yeasts) that live in and on our bodies.

Candida is usually a resident of the digestive system, mostly in the intestines. It also tends to occupy sites in the vaginal regions and on the skin.

Research has shown that almost everyone has antibodies to Candida. Truss states that Candida is evidenced by a positive skin test reaction when extracts of Candida are injected just under the skin.[2] The positive reaction shows that there has been a presence of the yeast for which the body has developed antibodies.

The fact that Candida is in all of us, and yet many people sail through life with no apparent ill effects, indicates that we have learned to cope with our passengers. Unlike certain other minute creatures that live in our digestive tract and serve a useful purpose, such as *lactobacillus acidophilus*, which helps with the breakdown of our food and in the synthesis of some of the B vitamins, Candida has no symbiotic relationship with our bodies. Candida is a freeloading parasite. It is perhaps inevitable that we should harbor such a parasite, considering the multitude of opportunistic microscopic creatures, of both the animal and vegetable kingdom. Most, if not all, plants and animals "enjoy" relationships with bacteria and fungi. Some of these relationships are mutually beneficial and some are distinctly one-sided. Candida, for all the musicality of its name, is an unwelcome boarder and a potential danger throughout our lives. Once we know just what sort of situations will remove our natural controls over it, and what environment will give it its extra ability to proliferate, we will have the beginnings of a picture of what we need to do to contain it.

Part of this picture is indeed an understanding of the ways in which the body meets the threat of parasites. We cannot actually stop Candida from taking up residence in our bodies, but we can certainly confine its activities to a small and relatively safe part of the premises.

Our bodies have amazing defensive capability. It has long been observed that people who survive certain infections seldom suffer from that same disease again. Apart from developing specific antibodies to resist various disease-causing microorganisms, the immune system plays a vital role in other biological reactions. We have, in essence, two systems that together make up the immune system. One is based in the thymus gland located just below the breast bone, which produces T cells. The other part of the immune system is made up of different types of white blood cells, called B cells. These protect you from most bacterial invaders and some viral infections. By producing molecules called antibodies, the B cells neutralize many potential enemies. The two systems, together making up the surveillance and protection agency of the body, work in harmony with, it is thought, the thymus gland taking the leading role.[3]

The white blood cells, which act as soldiers in the front line of the battle, are manufactured mainly in the marrow of the long bones of the body. Some of these actually turn into T cells, due to the influence of hormones from the thymus gland. Other white blood cells turn into lymphocytes. Anything that tries to get into the bloodstream, or the interior of the body, has to contend with the T and B cells and their powerful ability to neutralize foreign substances or organisms. If a B cell senses a foreign organism, it produces antibodies that are specific to that invader. At the same time, other B cells are alerted to the alien presence, which causes them to manufacture antibodies to destroy the enemy.

It is believed that there are in excess of a million different kinds of antibodies in the bloodstream. As they are manufactured and deployed against an intruder, the lymphocytes go into action with other white blood cells to dispose of the debris and waste products of the battle between the intruder and the body. Thus, a condition such as influenza is self-limiting, in that the fever and the symptoms of aching represent the intense body activity that is going on to handle the invading virus, as well as the effects resulting from the toxicity of the waste products of the battle.

When T cells come across an invading organism, whether it be a virus, or a fungus such as Candida (or even a mutant cancer cell), they produce lymphokines, which can kill microorganisms (and some cancer cells). One such lymphokine, which has received much attention, is interferon. Lymphokines can also call up assistance from a powerful ally, macrophage, which can eliminate microorganisms and tumor cells by literally swallowing them whole. Sometimes the T cells act as "helper" cells to the B cells in the production of antibodies to fight the invader, and they can also act as "suppressor" cells to stop a defensive process from getting out of hand, when there may be a danger of B or T cells actually attacking friendly tissues in the body.

When, for any one of a number of reasons, which we will consider in a later chapter, the immune system becomes weakened, we say that the person is immunodeficient, or has a poor immune response. It is when these valiant soldiers, the B and T cells, the macrophages, and their various assistants are in a weakened state that parasites in our body become free to spread to areas beyond their normal territory. At that point, a vast array of problems and symptoms can arise.

This system of defense, with its checks and balances, may become disrupted to such an extent that acquired immune deficiency syndrome (AIDS) may occur. In AIDS the T cells function inadequately. In fact, the ratio between the helper and suppressor cells alters so that there is an excess of suppressor cells, in contrast with the opposite ratio that exists in normal health. One research effort in the AIDS battle involves the use of thymosin, a hormone produced by the thymus gland. It is obviously desirable to enhance the function of the thymus gland so that it can produce enough active T cells and the desired amount of hormone. Among the nutrient factors that we can use to this end are vitamin C and the amino acid arginine. The amounts used in treating conditions, such as AIDS, where the immune system is severely disrupted, are very large indeed (up to 20 g of vitamin C daily, and 3 to 5 g of arginine).

When the immune system is in a weakened state, not only do infections become more frequent, but also severe consequences arise, such as greater likelihood of cancer developing, because of the reduced surveillance by the B and T cells. In such a condition of inadequate protection, it is no wonder that the ever present, opportunistic yeast may slip through the defense barrier and advance to areas previously closed to it. It is known that before Candida becomes invasive, it takes a different form, known as its mycelial fungal form, in which it has characteristics that make it more dangerous, such as a rootlike structure, enabling it to penetrate through mucosal barriers with a variety of harmful consequences (see Chapter 4, "Candida and Its Consequences to Your Health").

Recent research by Dr. Truss[35] indicates that many of the toxic effects of Candida activity result from its ability to manufacture, under appropriate conditions, the substance acetaldehyde. He points out that this well-known toxin could produce both the clinical and the laboratory characteristics of Candida infection. He has analyzed the amino acid profiles of affected individuals to arrive at this finding, and maintains that this theory appeals because it defines the symptoms of chronic yeast infection in terms of a toxin that common strains of Candida produce in laboratory conditions. This discovery provides the chemical link between normal yeast fermentation and the metabolic abnormalities found in susceptible patients. He stresses that no conclusive proof yet exists that Candida can ferment sugar into acetaldehyde in the body, but that this is highly probable, based on the evidence collected so far.

There is also evidence from a variety of sources[36, 37, 38] that a degree of immune system depression can result from mercury toxicity which can occur in the body because of amalgam fillings in the teeth. A number of researchers have shown that there are several ways in which this highly toxic metal is able to penetrate into the body, and that mercury has a specific harmful effect on the immune system. There is also evidence that mercury can be linked with the spread of Candida activity. A number of dentists are now helping affected individuals by removing mercury amalgams and replacing them with either a composite or gold filling. The research into the relationship between mercury and health problems in general, and Candida involvement in particular, is incomplete. Nevertheless, a link seems probable, and it is worth considering alternatives to amalgams, which contain mercury, for the filling for teeth. The replacement of existing fillings may be required in cases where a link can be demonstrated between one's health status and a measurable mercury toxicity, resulting from amalgams. The use of amino acid compounds, such as glutathione, and vitamin C can help to expel mercury deposits from the body. Tests can be conducted to measure the sensitivity of the body to mercury, and also to measure the levels of mercury in the mouth (escaping as a gas), as well as the electrical activity in the teeth that is caused by the combinations of metals in the mouth. These methods, as well as measuring mercury levels by hair analysis, can indicate how active this problem is in any particular individual.

Our attempt to neutralize and control the spread and effects of Candida (for we can seldom get rid of it completely) will involve using whatever safe methods we have at our disposal, to deprive it of its nutrients, while at the same time building up and enhancing the depleted immune system. It is this double thrust of effort that we must undertake if we are to get more than temporary results. The use of an antifungal drug will, in time, greatly reduce Candida's potency and alleviate negative symptoms. However, Candida returns in full force the moment the drug is stopped. Long term control of Candida requires a two-pronged attack that both deprives the yeast of its optimum environment and reinstates the immune system and beneficial intestinal flora. Other methods, it is thought, can also help lessen the ability of the yeast to multiply, and we will consider these natural, safe alternatives to drugs later.

It must be stated, however, that there are conditions in which the use of antifungal drugs are advocated (see Chapter 6, "Additional Methods of Candida Control"), especially if the process of recovery is going to be very long. For the most part, however, once we learn to recognize the symptoms that indicate that Candida is getting out of hand, the natural, non-drug methods that I am suggesting will work, and work well.

We will next consider just what can happen to weaken the immune system, as well as other changes that allow Candida to go on the rampage and infest other areas of your body.

3

How Candida Gets
Out of Hand

A number of predisposing factors will allow Candida to get wildly out of control. These factors may also be involved in the more subtle spread of Candida, represented by the kinds of symptoms described in Chapter 1. There is a degree of overlap, of course, for seldom is only one factor involved. The main factors are the following:

- An underlying inherited or acquired deficiency of the immune system.
- The aftermath of steroids (hormones) in food or as medication.
- The aftermath of antibiotics in food or as medication.
- Diabetes.

As we shall see, these factors are also vitally interconnected with our diet, which "feeds" the yeast. We will look at each of these factors to see how they help transform Candida from a relatively docile state into a predatory one. First, let us consider ways in which the immune system can be weakened.

Immune System Deficiency

As previously discussed, part of the body's response to an intruder such as Candida is to produce antibodies to combat the specific antigen that is present in the invading substance or organism. Candida has many antigens, and the efficiency with which the body's defensive operation is carried out against any particular one of these antigens can to some extent be inherited. There is great variation among people in their responses to different antigens. In some people, if the immune system is unable to adequately counteract and expel a Candida invasion, it tolerates the yeast in increasing amounts.

Research has demonstrated that we are all biochemically unique.[4, 5] This means that our requirements for any of the forty-plus nutrients needed for survival and health vary widely. Many individual needs are determined before birth, and this recognition has led to the genetotrophic theory of disease causation. Put simply, this theory says that because a person has individual, inborn requirements, which may vary greatly from a mythical norm, there is a good chance of one or another of these needs not being met by the normal diet. Deprivation leads at best to a lowered degree of function, and at worst to a deficiency disease.

To a large extent, the individual genetic factor also applies to our ability to handle any of the microorganisms that are capable of infecting us. This is the case with our ability to handle Candida efficiently. Some people will be more able than others to keep it under control and limit its spread. Thus, some people will, without such variables as antibiotics and steroid drugs, become somewhat "tolerant" of the spread of the yeast.

The most common areas for this spread to occur are the mouth, the throat, and the vagina. If the spread of Candida initially causes the immune system to react, then we would see a manifestation of a condition called thrush. This would flare up periodically when, perhaps, general vitality was lowered. Eventually, in many cases, the condition might no longer evoke an acute flare-up, but would remain in a chronic state. The body becomes "tolerant" of the yeast and is no longer able to attack it. This situation indicates an impaired or deficient immune function.

Among the many aspects of our environment that can lead to this result are stress, inadequate nutrition and pollution, as well as the use of drugs that further weaken the immune system. We are all familiar with the concept of tissue and organ transplantation. Transplants involve the use of powerful drugs designed to prevent the recipient's body from rejecting the new foreign tissue or organ. These are called immunosuppressive drugs, because their prime task is to stop the natural defenses from working. The risk of infection and of other diseases that results is all too familiar to patients who have gone through such treatment. Drugs such as steroids (hormones) also have this effect, and these are used for a variety of conditions, ranging from rheumatic disorders to asthma to hormonal imbalances. The most widespread use of steroids, however, is not in the treatment of disease but in the contraceptive pill. The long-term use of this type of medication can have a devastating effect on the immune system in general, and on the ability of Candida to proliferate unchecked, in particular.

We now know a variety of nutrients that are essential for the adequate functioning of the immune system.[6, 7] These include a number of vitamins and minerals that have antioxidant properties. They are able to slow down, or stop, a process in which substances known as "free radicals" can cause tissue damage. The major free-radical scavengers are vitamin C, vitamin E (acting in conjunction with selenium), as well as certain amino acids (parts of the protein chain) such as methionine, cysteine, and glutathione (which is itself a combination of three amino acids—cysteine, glutamic acid, and glycine). Deficiencies of vitamin B_6 (pyridoxine), zinc, manganese, and other important nutrients have been shown to be involved in compromising the immune system.[8]

Apart from the nutrients mentioned in this section, individual needs vary among people. One person may require extraordinary amounts of a particular nutrient due to heredity. Individual needs may also vary markedly under different conditions (infection, stress, pregnancy, and so on) in the same person, so any vitamin, mineral, or other nutrient deficiency is capable of upsetting the chain of complex biochemical interactions that allows the immune system to operate efficiently. The ones cited above just happen to have a more dramatic impact on the immune system than others. Assessment of personal needs requires patience. Some personal detective work can be useful, and books, such as *Your Personal Health Programme* by Jeffrey Bland and *Your Personal Vitamin Profile* by Michael Colgan, provide questionnaires to help you assess your own needs, that focus on specific nutritional requirements.

Stress, which involves repeated or constant states of anxiety, and the resulting depletion of vital nutrient reserves, as well as imbalances of internal secretions and functions, is a major cause of immune inadequacy. A dramatic demonstration of this is that during periods of stress people become far more prone to infection. The body's immune system efficiency is lowered, and the use of vital nutrients such as zinc and vitamin C is increased at such times.

If, at the same time, the demand on the immune system is increased, to meet environmental or nutritional toxicity (due to air pollution, cigarette smoke, alcohol, or caffeine-rich drinks such as coffee, chocolate, and tea), then a complex picture emerges in which excessive demands, inadequate nutrition (with associated deficiencies), and perhaps drug use (such as the contraceptive pill), all interact to further weaken the immune function. Let us examine the manner in which common drugs can further complicate the situation.

Antibiotics, "the Pill" and Steroids

Many years of research show that the use of antibiotics removes biological controls over Candida. One of the major sites where this can take place is the long, dark, warm, and moist (ideal environment for yeast) digestive tract, which is also inhabited by nearly five pounds of other microorganisms, most of which are friendly and helpful to the body. One such friend is lactobacillus acidophilus, which, by its presence, helps to keep a check on the spread of yeast. When antibiotics are used to destroy pathogenic microorganisms that are harming the body (as in treating an infection), the friendly bacteria in the digestive tract are also destroyed, or severely damaged. When this occurs, Candida, which is totally unaffected by the antibiotic (being a yeast and not a bacteria), finds room for expansion. Its spread becomes even more likely as the resistance of the immune system is also compromised at that time. In a variety of ways, the same thing happens with the use of steroid drugs such as cortisone (even cortisone ointments, so commonly prescribed for skin problems, can cause a yeast increase when they are absorbed into the system). All steroids, including those used in the contraceptive pill, have a depressing effect on the immune system.

It is worth noting that there is another, almost totally ignored source of antibiotics and hormonal residues, to which all but vegetarians are exposed. This is, of course, commercially produced meat (with the exception of lamb) and poultry. Antibiotics and hormones are fed to animals in order to speed their growth, as well as to control the heightened susceptibility to disease that their unnatural existence generates. Anyone who has been regularly eating beef, pork, veal, and chicken (and many people eat one or more of these daily) will have absorbed prodigious amounts of antibiotic and hormone residues (unless the source of the meat was a farm that does not use such drugs). Low-level intake of these drugs over many years may have a devastating effect on the ability to control Candida, as would the regular use of these substances in the form of medications. Although this area has yet to be adequately researched, it does provide one more argument in favor of a vegetarian diet.

Also, because of the hormonal changes that take place during pregnancy, a degree of control over Candida is lost during that time. Yeast, therefore, finds gestation a good time to expand its activities.

Imagine, then, a young woman who has grown up in this era, characterized by common use of drugs. She has had antibiotics pre-

scribed to her over the years for minor problems such as tonsillitis
and ear infection. She may have developed cystitis from time to time,
and also have taken a broad-spectrum antibiotic for that. She may have
had acne, which again would commonly have been treated with antibiotics. (Cystitis and acne are themselves often indications of Candida activity.) She may have had steroids for asthma or some other
condition. Going on "the Pill," then coming off it and becoming pregnant would also have enhanced the chances of yeast spreading and
causing problems. Thus, the child in her womb would be exposed to
a variety of antigens (up to 790) from the Candida activity in her body,
all the while inheriting the possibility of a weak immune response (not
all children inherit a weak response), allowing the pattern to repeat
itself. We have left out of this picture all the other variables, such as
nutritional imbalances (which are common in modern society), pollution, sugar-rich foods (which yeast loves), and stress. The picture
emerges of a person who is doing about all that is possible to bring
about the ideal conditions for Candida to thrive. And the result,
in terms of the general population, of this typical scenario? An
explosion of Candida-caused problems over the past thirty years or
so, which is now reaching epidemic proportions.

Truss, who has done so much to research and publicize the Candida problem, is scathing in his attack on the use of certain drugs that
compound the problem. Antibiotics are often used inadvisedly, in cases
in which they have no role to play at all. Incorrectly diagnosed viral
and fungal conditions may be uselessly treated with antibiotics, for
example. This actually increases the likelihood of the "treated" condition worsening. The treatment of acne with tetracycline is another
major cause of Candida spreading, and Truss insists that there is no
way that people suffering from Candida-caused problems can control
their condition if they continue taking tetracycline. In many cases, acne
is actually the direct result of Candida infection, and will worsen rather
than improve with such treatment.

In the use of the contraceptive pill, too, Truss sees great harm.

Fully 35 percent of the women using the Pill have, associated with it, acute vaginal candidiasis. There are undoubtedly many others who have less pronounced changes in this regard, as their immune competence is gradually compromised by the hormonal onslaught. As Truss points out, "Chronic yeast vaginitis tends to be at its worst when progesterone levels are high, as in pregnancy and the luteal phase of the menstrual cycle. Therefore, the progesterone component of contraceptive hormones may well be responsible for their effect." Moreover, an association between Candida vaginitis and emotional problems, such as irritability and depression, frequently appears soon after the first use of the contraceptive pill. It is worth reflecting on the fact that the degree of biological individuality that we display in our reactions to harmful invaders must play a large part in determining who is, and who is not, susceptible to a spread of Candida. Since 35 percent of women do suffer from vaginal candidiasis when on the Pill, we must assume that the other 65 percent do not. This highlights the fact that many people have an inborn genetic weakness in their ability to meet such a challenge.

Controlling Candida must include methods that deal both with the building up of the immune system, as well as reducing the means that sustain the yeast in its advance. Among the most important of these is the elimination (unless absolutely vital) of antibiotics, hormonal preparations, and contraceptive pills, as well as alterations in the diet to avoid feeding the yeast.

Foods That Help to Spread Candida

Yeast loves carbohydrate-rich foods. This in effect means that we must attempt to deprive it of its sustenance by limiting, or cutting out all together, all sugar-rich foods and refined carbohydrates. Because yeast loves sugar, it is clear that additional levels of sugar in the bloodstream, as in a diabetic condition, will fuel the spread of Candida. For this reason diabetic individuals are more prone to Candida problems, and they must be even more rigorous in their efforts to control it.

The possible involvement of mercury toxicity in harming immune system control of Candida has been mentioned (see page 21) and deserves re-emphasis. It is also important to limit the intake of any foods that contain fermented products, molds, or fungi.[2, 9] Included are vinegar, alcoholic beverages, yeast extracts and spreads, mushrooms, and blue cheeses. Avoidance of certain foods to control Candida should be carefully observed at first, but once the yeast is controlled, there is no reason to keep to a strict abstinence. The return of the classic symptoms of Candida activity, such as abdominal bloating after eating one of the offending foods, will tell you if it is time to return for a period to the avoidance strategy.

Just as foods that contain molds or fungi are undesirable, so are humid, damp environments, which support mold and fungus spores in the atmosphere. Thus, it is important to eliminate from the home any damp areas. Molds can reinforce the effects of Candida by their presence. For this reason, avoid inhaling spores of any mold or fungus during the active phase of Candida infection.

Candida gets out of hand because we allow it to. We may do so in ignorance, but it is foolish to blame the yeast when we have the power to control it. Once you suspect that your symptoms may be the result of Candida activity, it is time to take responsibility for the situation. Candida will not go away. Its current spree may be the result of any combination of factors that have released it from our normal efficient control. To get it back where it belongs (or at least where it can do least harm) we must restore our defense capacity to its optimum, and we must stop doing those things that are helping the yeast to thrive. It's as simple as that. You can do this by your own efforts, by changing your diet, by using appropriate nutritional supplements, and by reducing overall stress and pollution. Once you have put Candida in its place, you can relax your vigilance to a great extent, in the sense of allowing your diet to contain some of the "undesirable" foods from time to time; still, you should be aware of the conditions that allow Candida to advance in the first place, and avoid them as stringently as possible.

Next, we'll look at the symptoms that Candida can cause when it gets out of control. Be prepared for some surprises!

4

Candida and Its Consequences for Your Health

The list of physical problems in which Candida has been implicated as a major causative factor is very long indeed.

It is useless to ask a microbiology lab to look for Candida because we already know it is present in practically all adults. We must deduce from the person's history and the symptoms that Candida is causing a problem. (Were antibiotics used? Is, or was, the contraceptive pill used? Have cortisones or other steroids, such as prednisone, been used? And so on.) The range and type of symptoms also indicate its involvement. The proof is obtained by carrying out an anti-Candida program and seeing if most of the symptoms disappear.

Before considering the major symptoms, one by one, let us look at a list of the conditions that are now known to be the possible result of Candida's activity:

Vaginitis; thrush (oral or vaginal); endometriosis; athlete's foot; headaches (migraine type); fatigue; constipation; bloating; allergy; sensitivity to perfumes, fumes, chemical odors and tobacco smoke; poor memory; feelings of unreality; irritability; inability to concentrate; depression; numbness; tingling and weak muscles; heart-burn; abdominal pain; diarrhea; recurring sore throat and nasal congestion; swelling and discomfort in joints; blurred vision; and so on—and on. The diagnosis becomes even more clear if the symptoms are aggravated by damp weather (or places) or by an environment with a lot of mold or fungus. Also, if the symptoms are worse after eating sugar-rich or fungus-containing foods, the evidence for Candida's involvement becomes stronger.

Truss draws a picture of a typical case of chronic Candida infection in his article "Restoration of Immunological Competence to Candida Albicans."[10] He states, after pointing out effects of multiple pregnancies, birth control pills, antibiotics, and cortisone, as well as other factors that depress the immune system:

> The onset of local symptoms of yeast infection, in relation to the use of these drugs, is especially significant and usually precedes the systemic response. Repeated courses of antibiotics and birth-control pills, often punctuated with multiple pregnancies, lead to ever increasing symptoms of mucosal infections in the vagina and gastrointestinal tract. Accompanying these are manifestations of tissue injury, based on immunological and possibly toxic responses to yeast products released into the systemic circulation. Many infections are secondary to allergic responses of the mucous membranes of the respiratory tract, urethra and bladder, necessitating increasingly frequent antibiotic therapy that simultaneously aggravates, and perpetuates, the underlying cause of the allergic membrane, that allowed the infection. Depression is common, often associated with difficulty in memory, reasoning and concentration. These symptoms are especially severe in women, who in addition have great difficulty with the explosive irritability, crying and loss of self-confidence that are so characteristic of abnormal function of the ovarian hormones.

Truss then points out that accompanying this sad catalog is what he calls "poor end-organ response" which results in acne; loss of libido (disinterest in sex); menstrual bleeding and cramps; intolerance to foods and chemicals; and so on. Commonly, the people who suffer from Candida infection are women between puberty and menopause, who have a history of some, or all, of the predisposing factors described previously, and who have some, or all, of the symptoms outlined in Truss's picture above. A combination of unaccountable vaginal and bowel problems, ranging from discharge and itching, to bloating, discomfort, diarrhea and/or constipation, as well as an array of mental and emotional symptoms are typical. Classically such women are labeled neurotic—the crowning insult to a person who has literally begun to feel her body and mind giving way in all directions.

If circumstances allow, Candida can spread along the entire length of the digestive tract, from the anus to the mouth. The tongue may be coated, and there may be yeast deposits on the insides of the cheeks, the corners of the mouth, and the gums. White spots and a coating on the tongue, accompanied by a soreness and tingling of the gums, are the obvious signs. When the esophagus is affected, it can result in symptoms commonly dismissed as "heartburn." Indigestion and acid stomach are symptoms that can be the result of Candida activity in the stomach. If the infestation is prolific in the small or large intestine, diarrhea may be the result. This condition may be chronic, and may be accompanied by mucus and/or blood. There may be cramplike pains ("spastic colon") and colicky pains, often associated with difficult bowel movements. Bloating and distension of the abdomen is a frequent occurrence with Candida, and there may be a variety of abdominal noises as a result. If constipation is indeed a factor, then hemorrhoids are a likely consequence, as is the possibility of rectal discomfort and itching.

As I've mentioned, Candida is a dimorphic organism, meaning that it has two separate identities: a yeast form and a fungal form. In the yeast form, it has no root; but in its fungal form, it produces rhizoids—long rootlike structures. These "roots" can actually penetrate the mucosa of the tissue in which they are growing, and can thus breach the boundary between the body proper and the self-contained world of the digestive tract. Substances that would otherwise have been kept out by this boundary can then enter the bloodstream. The invasive fungal form of Candida can use this means to enter the body proper. The serious result of the penetration of the intestinal barrier is that undigested proteins from food, as well as toxic wastes from the Candida infestation, may begin to circulate in the bloodstream. These frequently cause a wide variety of disseminated symptoms, often of an allergic type. If these substances reach the brain, there is a chance that "brain allergies will develop".[11] These can result in a wide variety of mood and personality problems, ranging from depression, irritability, and mood swings to symptoms that resemble schizophrenia.

These errant substances, which enter the brain and act on the receptors there, producing negative mental and personality symptoms, have been labeled *exorphins*.[12] This differentiates them from *endorphins*, which are substances produced by the body to help in the control of many aspects of the biochemistry of life, including pain control. The externally originating substances (proteins from incompletely digested food) that slip into the bloodstream through the passages made by fungal "roots" of Candida can cause havoc in any tissues they contact. They are "foreign" to the immune system, which will attempt to neutralize them. If this neutralization process is continued for long (this sort of thing can go on for many years), then this in itself is a factor contributing to the ultimate depletion of the immune system of the body. The system simply becomes overwhelmed by the constant onslaught. The defensive reaction by the immune system to such substances may result in a wide range of what are seen as allergic symptoms, including asthmatic attacks, nasal and respiratory conditions, skin reactions, palpitations, aches, swellings, and so on.

The female reproductive organs are another major site for Candida activity. Irritation of the urethra can be a common cause of cystitis. If, for any of a number of reasons, the acidity of the region changes, Candida's relatively benign yeast form can change into the fungal form and become actively invasive, spreading to other regions accessible from the vagina. This can lead to inflammatory conditions in the womb, fallopian tubes, and ovaries. A wide variety of consequences can be envisaged, including the possibility of infertility or sterility. The symptoms related to Candida involvement in this region may range from frequency of urination, coupled with a burning sensation, to chronic discharge, as well as premenstrual and menstrual problems, and the whole gamut of inflammatory and infectious involvements of the reproductive system.

The concurrence of mild, or major, emotional and mental symptoms with any of the described patterns of ill health should alert you to the strong possibility of Candida activity. Often, the mental symptoms are no more than a general feeling of inability to concentrate, accompanied by memory lapses, and feelings of lethargy and exhaustion. They may, however, be far more dramatic, as Truss and others have shown. The first articles on the subject, by Truss, discussed the fact that many conditions are given names or "labels" because they fit into a pattern that somewhat resembles a known illness. That is to say, a combination of symptoms that may have no obvious cause is somehow more "manageable" medically if it is labeled.

Truss initially reported six cases, all of them women. Two of these women had been repeatedly diagnosed as schizophrenic; another had been diagnosed as having multiple sclerosis. Pointing out that they all recovered on anti-yeast treatment and that they were all in good health up to seventeen years after recovery, Truss asked "Were two of these women really schizophrenic, or was it just that Candida albicans was responsible for brain function so abnormal that highly competent specialists never doubted the diagnosis of schizophrenia?" He further asked, "In the third woman, did Candida albicans induce neurological abnormalities sufficiently typical of multiple sclerosis that a competent neurologist would mistakenly diagnose the disease?" He concluded that either a yeast infection could produce symptoms that mimic these diseases (and many others), or the yeast could actually cause the diseases that are labeled with these names. The indication, after many years of work by Truss and others, is that these recoveries were not just cases of remission (which is not uncommon in either schizophrenia or multiple sclerosis), but that Candida induces symptoms similar to those of other illnesses, which may then be wrongly diagnosed and labeled.

Clearly, the ramifications of Candida infection are not yet fully understood, and much clarification and research remains to be done. In the meantime, because it is not difficult to identify reasons to suspect its possible involvement, it seems reasonable that a Candida-control approach should be adopted in cases where the history and symptoms approximate any of the patterns touched on above, whatever previous diagnosis has been made. The treatment is, after all, harmless and indeed health-promoting.

Other conditions that are sometimes caused by Candida are frequently labeled as psychosomatic. Doctors can thus avoid having to say that they cannot find the cause. Calling these conditions "functional" or "psychosomatic" may result in patients beginning to believe that it is all in their heads. The terms "neurotic" and "nervous" are often ascribed to people with devastating effects on morale and self-esteem. The yeast or fungal cause may remain unsuspected or, if noted as part of the problem (if thrush is part of the "psychosomatic" symptom picture, for example), may be simply ignored as a minor piece of the puzzle, unworthy of therapeutic effort.

We have reason to believe that Candida infection is rampant in modern society. It has been let loose by the use of drugs (used in good faith to help people), as well as by a diet that is ideal for the yeast, rather than the host. The number and variety of possible consequences is mind-boggling and deserves the attention of everyone involved in the healing professions.

Truss's alertness has brought about the current increased awareness of the significance of Candida. He may not be totally right in his concept, but the results he has so far obtained in the thousands of cases exhibiting a range of symptoms such as those already discussed—simply by paying attention to the yeast component of the problem—prove the validity of his method of treatment.

There is no health problem more amenable to self-assessment and self-help than cases in which Candida is the culprit. The checklists on the following pages will give you the chance to assess the possibility that Candida is a major part of your current health picture. It is possible for most of the symptoms described to be the result of causes other than Candida. If, however, you answer "yes" to more than one of the symptoms on List 2, as well as some of the lesser symptoms listed at the end of the list, the possibility that Candida is involved increases to a probability, especially if you can identify a possible link with at least one of the factors in List 1.

Candida Albicans Checklist

Answers to these questions will give clues as to whether Candida is an active agent in your current health picture. It is not possible to make a diagnosis by this means alone, but positive answers in all sections of the questionnaire are a strong indication. The results can assist you in deciding to undertake the Candida-control program.

List 1: History of Medications and Pregnancy

1. Have you ever taken antibiotics for an infection for a period of eight weeks or longer, or for short periods four or more times in one year?
2. Have you ever taken antibiotics for the treatment of acne for a period of a month or more?
3. Have you ever taken steroids such as predisone, cortisone, or ACTH?
4. Have you ever taken contraceptive pills for a year or more?
5. Have you ever been treated with immunosuppressant medications?

6. Have you been pregnant more than once?

List 2: History of Major Symptoms Implicating Candida

1. Have you had recurrent or persistent cystitis, vaginitis, or prostatitis?
2. Have you had a history of endometriosis?
3. Have you had thrush (oral or vaginal) more than once?
4. Have you ever had athlete's foot or a fungal infection of the nails or skin?
5. Are you severely affected by exposure to chemical fumes, perfumes, tobacco smoke, and so on? Or are your symptoms worse after taking yeasty or sugary foods or drinks?
6. Do you suffer from a variety of allergies?
7. Do you commonly suffer from abdominal distension, "bloating," diarrhea, or constipation?
8. Do you suffer from premenstrual syndrome (fluid retention, irritability, and so on)?
9. Do you suffer from depression, fatigue, lethargy, poor memory, or feelings of "unreality"?
10. Do you crave sweet foods, bread, or alcohol?
11. Do you suffer from unaccountable muscle aches, tingling, numbness, or burning?
12. Do you suffer from unaccountable aches and swelling in the joints?
13. Do you have a vaginal discharge or irritation, or menstrual cramps or pain?
14. Do you have erratic vision or spots before the eyes?
15. Do you suffer from impotence or lack of sexual desire?

If you answer "yes" to one or more questions in the first section and to two or more in the second section, and some of the following symptoms are present, then Candida is probably involved in your symptoms: Symptoms ususally worse on damp days; persistent drowsiness; lack of coordination; headaches; mood swings; loss of balance; rashes; mucus in stools; belching and flatulence; bad breath; postnasal drip; nasal itch and/or congestion; nervous irritability; tightness in the chest; dry mouth or throat; ear sensitivity or fluid in the ears; and heartburn and indigestion.

5

Controlling Candida Naturally

If you believe that Candida is a likely suspect in your health problem, you can test your supposition by following an anti-Candida program. If your condition greatly improves and your symptoms abate, you will have proved your assumption to be correct. Dr. W.M. Crook calls this a "therapeutic trial."[9] It is really the only way of being sure, because there is as yet no laboratory test to prove that Candida is involved.

This clinical uncertainty is a stumbling block for many people. They want absolute "proof" that Candida is the culprit. However, all we can do is look at the current picture of your particular condition and add to this a review of your past history. If the combination looks like a "Candida picture," then the best choice is to begin anti-Candida measures. If a culture were made of your fluid discharges, tissues, or feces, it would inevitably indicate Candida's presence somewhere in your body. This would not prove or disprove anything as far as your symptoms are concerned, because a positive test result could also be obtained from almost every adult in the world. Only by looking at the known and suspected pattern of symptoms can we suspect Candida's active presence (as opposed to its benign presence, which results when your immune system and intestinal flora are keeping it under control). The very least that you will achieve in following the anti-Candida program is that you will have reformed your diet, and will have swallowed some harmless vitamins and other supplements, as well as building up your immune system's ability to combat its adversaries.

A control program for Candida has three components. First, there are a number of nutritional supplements that, for several reasons, can help to control Candida. Second, there is a pattern of eating that reduces the intake of yeast supporting foods, depriving it of its growth potential. Finally, there are special methods and substances, including antifungal drugs, that can be prescribed only by a licensed physician. The third category will be discussed to complete the picture of anti-Candida methods, although, as we have stressed, it is in self-help that the greatest long-term results will be found. The first two components of the program, special supplements and diet, will prove worth of adoption by people suspicious of Candida's role in their current health picture.

Anti-Candida Agents

Antibiotics destroy a number of "friendly" bacteria that inhabit the digestive tract and provide other valuable symbiotic (mutually beneficial) benefits to the body while also stopping Candida from spreading. One of our major bacterial "friends" is lactobacillus acidophilus. Taking acidophilus is an important element in this program. If a sufficient number of this bacteria can be encouraged to re-establish residence in the bowel, they will push back the yeast, which may have crowded into the vacant space left when antibiotics destroyed acidophilus colonies. Lactobacillus acidophilus is obtainable in a number of forms. It comes in capsules and also, in its active state, in some yogurt cultures. Cultured milk products containing acidophilus should therefore play a part in the anti-Candida program.

A number of sources and types of acidophilus are worth mentioning. A recent development in the US is "Megadophilus." One of the 200-plus strains of lactobacillus acidophilus has been identified by Natasha Trenev, a research authority in the field of cultured dairy produce, as being infinitely more potent in its ability to destroy undesirable bacteria, than other strains. Her discovery has been incorporated into "Megadophilus," which contains at least one billion active organisms per gram. This is over a hundred times more potent than comparable commercial acidophilus preparations and, in some cases, many thousands of times more potent. Some researchers have found that acidophilus cultured in human milk is more effective than that cultured in animal milk, and the human milk technique is believed to be that used in the manufacture of Megadophilus. This and another similar product, "Vital Dophilus," should be the first choices in acidophilus supplementation (see "Further Information" for suppliers). Dosage of either Megadophilus or Vital Dophilus, as dry powder or as a capsule, is 2 g (or one teaspoon) three times daily between meals. Dosages of up to 10 g (five teaspoons of powder) daily are in order with no toxic level known. If in powder form, the acidophilus should be kept refrigerated and never exposed to temperatures above 80°F. When consumed as a powder, it should be stirred into unchilled water and drunk. The acidophilus culture will become active in the small intestine, where it produces a number of nutritional compounds, including lactic acid, B vitamins, and enzymes, as well as natural antibiotic compounds.[13, 14, 15]

In the average bowel, there exist colonies of microorganisms that weigh a total of between three and five pounds. These are not all helpful or friendly, and in order to repopulate the bowel with such helpful residents as acidophilus, large amounts of it are required. As benign bacteria re-establish their territorial claim, intruders like Candida will be pushed back and often eliminated from the area. Megadophilus between meals, then, is the first of the anti-Candida supplements you should use, together with acidophilus-cultured yogurt and/or milk with meals.

The next major nutrient you can use against Candida is the B vitamin biotin, also called vitamin H. Research in Japan has indicated a fascinating way in which Candida can be deterred from changing from its relatively harmless yeast form into its invasive and dangerous fungal form.[17] The change of form is found to occur more rapidly in a medium in which there is a relative biotin deficiency. Biotin deficiency in humans results in a number of skin conditions. These include a dermatitis that is characterized by a grayish, dry, flaky appearance. This is accompanied by a lack of appetite, nausea, lassitude, and muscular pains. It is interesting to note that all of these symptoms are common when Candida is proliferating, and it is worth questioning whether the supposed symptoms of biotin deficiency are not at least in part the result of Candida activity, brought about by that deficiency.

Egg white contains a substance called avidin, which is capable of combining with biotin, thus neutralizing its usefulness in the body. For this reason, raw egg should not be included in the anti-Candida diet (avidin is destroyed by cooking).

Biotin should be taken as a supplement, three times daily, in doses of 350 to 500 mcg with acidophilus between meals.

Another anti-Candida agent is garlic, which has been the subject of research worldwide. Russian scientists have proved its long-reputed antibacterial quality by the introduction of garlic extract into colonies of bacteria, which ceased to function within minutes. Fresh garlic juice was used in these tests. Reports in Western medical and scientific journals confirm such claims,[18] in this case against salmonella typhimurium and escherichia coli, two extremely active microorganisms. Garlic is also active against yeast and fungi. This was confirmed in recent reports that showed it to be more active against human ringworm (a fungal infection) than currently used drugs.[19] *The Book of Garlic* (Thorsons, U.K.) quotes a researcher as stating, "Garlic in the form of juice is a very potent anti-microbial agent, both to bacteria, and pathogenic yeasts. We can thus suppose, at least, that staphylococcal, fungal skin, and alimentary tract disease can be effectively cured by the juice of garlic."[20]

Research at the University of Indiana suggests that the value of garlic against fungal infections is very great. "An aqueous extract of garlic bulbs inhibits growth of many aspects of zoopathogenic fungi," the first report stated.[21] The second concluded, "Allicin (the active sulphur-rich compound in garlic) may provide the model system for chemotherapy of candida albicans infections."[22]

The gastronomic aspect of garlic is, of course, a factor to consider. While many people can happily eat whole cloves of garlic, others find the taste and odor unpleasant. For them, the recent development of a completely odorless garlic (Kyolic) is a boon (see "Futher Information" for suppliers).

Part of the anti-Candida campaign should include the daily intake of either fresh or deodorized garlic in capsule form. The former is preferred; the latter is an acceptable compromise. Take two to three garlic capsules, morning and evening, after meals, or eat as much raw garlic as you can learn to enjoy. Slice it finely on cooked vegetables, or press it on salads, or simply eat it, clove by clove, with fish or poultry, as many Greeks do.

A further aid in the prevention of the transformation of Candida to its fungal form is olive oil.[16] This oil contains oleic acid, which acts on the yeast in a way similar to biotin. The recommended amount of olive oil is six teaspoons daily, divided into three doses. This can be included with meals or taken before or after, as desired.

Supplements for Immune-System Enhancers

In order to strengthen the immune system, it is suggested that a number of vitamins be included in the anti-Candida program. The primary nutrient is vitamin C. We have discussed this vitamin's importance in the economy of the body and its defensive T cells, which contain a very high level of vitamin C. It has been noted that the lower the vitamin C content of these vital cells, the less efficient is their performance in defending the body against intruding organisms or materials.[6, 7] This is a water-soluble vitamin, and the body does not store it, so a constant supply is needed. Any stress factor, pollutant, or infection puts demands on the vitamin C in the body. Research has shown that a fascinating adaptation takes place when requirements increase because of such factors as these. Under normal conditions, if people take more vitamin C than they actually need, they are likely to develop a degree of diarrhea. If someone takes 5 g daily with no diarrhea resulting, then it can be assumed that he or she needs that amount at that time. If under normal conditions, however, he or she develops diarrhea after ingesting only 2 g daily, it can be shown that should circumstances change and the need for vitamin C increase due to infection, stress, or some other factor, then that same person could increase his or her vitamin C intake by many times the previous tolerance level, without any bowel symptoms at all. Dr. Robert Cathcart has shown that, if necessary, the intake of vitamin C can be as high as 100 g a day (never try this without supervision) with no apparent bowel sensitivity.[23] When the crisis passes, however, such high doses do produce diarrhea, as previously. Thus the body, in its wisdom, is able to alter its normal way of functioning to meet specific requirements.

In order to assist a deficient immune system that might accompany a Candida spread, the recommended amount of vitamin C (in the absence of any bowel reaction) is 1 to 3 g daily, with food.

The effect of vitamin C on the T cells depends, of course, on the T cells being there to do their work. The thymus gland can become relatively inactive, and one of the main nutrients that can enhance its production of T cells is the amino acid arginine.[24] A dose of 3 g daily for a short period (say a month) will boost the thymus activity at the outset of the anti-Candida program, when it is most needed.

Note: If there is a history of herpes simplex infection, do not take arginine supplementally, for it has also been found to enhance herpes activity (this activity is countered by another amino acid, lysine).[25]

Take the arginine on an empty stomach, with water, before retiring. A long-term use of arginine at these levels is not suggested, although there are no known side effects in doses lower than 20 g daily. Rough, thickened skin may develop on the elbows, for example, in doses above 20 g daily, but this will disappear when the supplementation is stopped. The reason for suggesting a time limit to the use of arginine is that the thymus may come to depend upon such nutritional supplementation, instead of being encouraged to return to normal activity by the total program of Candida suppression. Therefore, take 3 g daily for only the first month of this program.

A further aid to the immune system is to increase the intake of certain B vitamins.[6] It is important that these not be derived from yeast sources.[2, 9] All the B vitamins are available in synthetic forms and these rather than yeast-derived vitamins, are suggested in cases involving Candida. Between 20 and 50 mg of vitamin B_6 (pyridoxine), between 20 and 50 mcg of vitamin B_{12}, and the same quantity of folic acid should be taken daily.

An additional B vitamin, B_5, should also be taken to enhance the B lymphocytes, especially if there is any evidence of allergic reactions or digestive involvement. This should be taken in the form of calcium pantothenate, at a dose of 500 mg daily.

The minerals zinc, selenium, and magnesium are all also commonly implicated in deficient immune response conditions,[5, 6, 11] and should ideally be added to the program. Just as in the selection of B vitamins, it is important to obtain selenium from a non-yeast source. This may prove difficult, but if there is sufficient demand, supply will increase. Dosages for specific minerals are as follows: zinc (in the form of zinc orotate), 50 mg daily; selenium, 50 mcg daily; and magnesium, 250 to 500 mg daily. All should be taken with food.

Finally, some of the fat-soluble vitamins are needed in our effort to resuscitate the immune response. These include a moderate intake of vitamin E (make sure that you are buying natural vitamin E, which can be identified by the name *d*-alpha tocopherol, rather than *dl*-alpha tocopherol, a synthetic form), in a dose of around 200IU daily; vitamin A in the form of beta carotene, in a dose of around 10,000IU daily; and finally, oil of evening primrose (vitamin F), in a 500 mg capsule twice daily.

Summary of Supplements

Anti-Candida Agents

Lactobacillus acidophilus: 2 g one to three times daily, between meals (Megadophilus or Vital Dophilus for preference).
Biotin (vitamin H): 350 to 500 mcg with acidophilus, three times daily.
Garlic capsules (if lots of fresh garlic is not being eaten as part of the regular diet): Three capsules, twice daily (morning and evening), after meals (Kyolic recommended—deodorized form).
Oleic acid (virgin, first-pressing olive oil): 2 teaspoons three times daily. Can be taken with meals or separately.

Immune-System Enhancers

Vitamin C: 1 g three times daily, with meals.
Arginine: 3 g with water, on an empty stomach, before retiring. Take for one month only.
Vitamin B_6 (pyridoxine): 20 to 50 mg daily.   Or one vitamin B-
Vitamin B_{12}: 20 to 50 mcg daily.   complex capsule
Folic acid: 20 to 50 mcg daily.   (yeast free) daily
Calcium pantothenate (B5): 500 mg daily (especially if allergy symptoms present).
Selenium: 50 mcg daily.
Zinc: 50 mg daily.
Magnesium: 250 to 500 mg daily.
Vitamin E (d-alpha tocopherol): 200IU daily.
Vitamin A (as beta carotene): 10,000IU daily.

Vitamin F (as oil of evening primrose): one or two 500 mg capsules daily.

Note: Ensure vitamin C is "with bioflavinoids"; ensure that B vitamins and selenium are not from a yeast source; ensure that zinc and magnesium are in orotate form (B-13 zinc, and B-13 magnesium).

It is clear from this discussion that we are using supplements to fight Candida on two fronts at the same time. First, we are using acidophilus and biotin (as well as oleic acid) to directly inhibit the alteration of Candida into its dangerous fungal form, and to resist its spread. Second, we are using the other nutrients to build up the immune function (B and T cells) so that the body can better cope with the invading microorganism. This two-pronged attack requires that you take this large number of supplements at the same time, which is both moderately expensive and unappealing. Let it be clear, however, that what is at stake is your health. For this reason, there should be no hesitation in grasping the opportunity to fight off the cause of your ill health by whatever safe methods are at hand. The methods advocated here are safe. They are also effective in most cases. It takes time to control Candida once it is rampant, and six months should be seen as the minimum length of time to maintain this program.

Our next consideration is the importance of combining the supplemental attack on Candida and the enhancement of the immune system with a diet that deprives the yeast of its main sources of food.

Anti-Candida Diet

There are two major areas to consider in the diet necessary to reduce the spread and activity of Candida. The first is the elimination of all foods derived from, or containing, yeasts or fungi. The second is the reduction, as far as possible, of all carbohydrate-rich foods, in order to deprive Candida of its favorite nourishment, which as anyone who has made beer or wine will testify, is sugar.

Foods Derived from or Containing
Fungi and Yeast

Foods and substances that contain yeast or yeast-like substances should be avoided as much as possible during the initial stages of dealing with Candida infection. It is wise to abstain from these foods for at least three months, after which time you can relax a little with the proviso that if such foods are reintroduced, and symptoms that had become quiescent become active again, a return to a stricter mode of eating, for a time, is called for. The rationale behind such avoidance is that in practice these foods seem to aggravate a Candida-induced condition, especially if allergic symptoms are part of the picture, as well as if there are symptoms such as bloating and intestinal gas.[2, 9] In a letter Truss states:

> If someone has no symptoms, I see no reason to have him avoid these yeast promoting foods, although I will say that in excess, and combined with a high-carbohydrate intake [sugars, etc.], these may actually induce this condition [Candida infection] even without the stimulatory effects of antibiotics, birth control pills, cortisone, etc.

The following foods contain yeast as an added ingredient in their preparations,[26] and are therefore undesirable, especially in the early stages of an anti-Candida program.

- Breads (non-yeasted whole wheat or corn bread is acceptable).
- Cakes and cake mixes.
- Cookies and crackers.
- Enriched flour.
- Buns, rolls, and pastries.
- Anything fried in breadcrumbs (fish sticks, etc.).

The following contain yeast, or yeast-like substances, because of the nature of their manufacture, or of their own nature.

- Mushrooms.
- Truffles.

- Soy sauce.
- Buttermilk and sour cream.
- Black tea.
- All cheeses, including cottage cheese.
- Citric acid (almost always a yeast derivative).
- Citrus drinks if canned or frozen.
- All dried fruits.
- All fermented beverages, such as beer, spirits, wine, cider, and ginger ale.
- All malted products (cereals, sweets, or dairy products that have been malted).
- All foods containing monosodium glutamate (which is often a yeast derivative).
- All vinegars, whether grape, malt, cider, or anything else. These are frequently used in sauces and relishes, as well as salad dressings, sauerkraut, olives, and pickled foods.

The following are either derived from yeast, or contain elements that are.

- Antibiotics.
- Multivitamin tablets (unless specifically stating that they are from a non-yeast source).
- B-complex vitamins (unless specifically stating that they are from a non-yeast source).
- Selenium (as above).
- Individual B vitamins (as above).

Truss singles out some foods from this long list as the main culprits. He states: "It is my belief that there are several foods that are primarily to be avoided. These include all fermented drinks, as well as vinegar, mushrooms, and moldy cheeses. I allow my patients to have cottage cheese, as well as yogurt." He goes on further to say, "It is rational to remove all of these foods from the diet only if there is an indication that the patients are having trouble with yeast (Candida)."[27]

In this light, it should be clear that the elimination of all alcoholic beverages and vinegar (and food prepared with vinegar, as listed) as well as the foregoing of the joys of blue cheeses and the eating of mushrooms, are the major areas of change for several months.

Sugar-Rich Foods

Sugar (sucrose) itself, in whatever guise, is to be strictly avoided during the battle to control Candida. This means white sugar, brown sugar, black sugar, and any shade in between. There is no such thing as a healthful sugar. We do not need sugar for health, and its sole attraction is its taste, which it is quite easy to do without. All sugar will aid the growth and proliferation of yeast. This includes syrups, honey (yes, I'm afraid so), and other forms of sugar, such as fructose, maltose, glucose, sorbitol, and so on. It includes molasses, date sugar, maple sugar, and all of that range of non-foods with which our real foods and beverages have been sweetened. Candy, chocolates, and all soft drinks should also be totally avoided.

Honey may come as a surprise to you in this context. I myself had assumed that honey was relatively safe, in that it did not seem, to my knowledge, to become moldy. I was corrected by Dr. Truss, who explained that honey does indeed contain yeast spores. He pointed out, "Species of zygosaccharomyces [a yeast] have been found particularly active in causing yeast spoilage of honey." It is known that honey is indeed hygroscopic (it absorbs water) and that at a certain degree of moisture content, there will be sufficient water at the surface to lower the concentration of sugars to a point that the yeasts and bacteria that might be present, can grow. Thus yeasts and other microorganisms that are capable of surviving in concentrated sugar solutions (in which no yeast will grow) become, at a certain point in the dilution of that medium, able to thrive. In order to prevent this from happening, honey is heated and often has additives, such as sodium benzoate, to inhibit the growth of fermenting yeasts. Truss and Crook both insist that honey be added to the list of banned foods during the anti-Candida campaign, and this is also my view. The length of time that this will be necessary will depend upon the rate of recovery. You should not expect it to be less than three months, and it is more likely to be six.

The most important single dietary alteration that the Candida sufferer can make is to eliminate sugar-rich foods from the diet.

As has already been discussed, the undesirability of eating foods containing yeast during recovery removes from the diet bread, pastry, cookies, cakes, and so on. This is doubly necessary, since these are mainly undesirable because of their high carbohydrate content (unless totally whole grain).

Any carbohydrate which has been refined beyond the simple grinding stage is undesirable. Whole wheat, oats used in cooked cereal, millet, and brown rice are all highly desirable foods, rich in what are known as complex carbohydrates. These can and indeed should (especially oats) be a part of the diet. Once these are broken down into fine flours and are refined further, they become less desirable, and actually become food for the yeast, rather than for you.

So even in the middle stages of the anti-Candida program when, hopefully, symptoms are on the wane and you might justifiably feel that a little relaxation of the stricter aspects of the diet are allowable, please remember that refined carbohydrates are the natural food of yeast, and Candida will thank you for the delivery of such foods by a rapid increase in its activity. As Truss puts it, "Decreased availability of carbohydrates slows the rate of multiplication of yeast cells, and thus should reduce the amount of yeast products entering the blood stream." The converse is true as well: the more of these foods there are in the diet, the greater will the chances be of further spread of Candida. So out of the diet goes pasta, pastry, flour products of all sorts, cookies, cakes, buns, rolls, bread (unless any of these are made with whole grains and without yeast or sugar).

Many foods have "hidden sugar," in that sugar is added in the processing or preparation. These are often foods with which sugar is not usually associated. Frozen peas, most canned foods, and many packaged and processed foods, all contain either refined flour products or sugar, or both. For this reason, as well as for the general undesirability of many such foods from a nutritional viewpoint, these should be avoided. Not only are you actually providing the favorite foods of the yeasts within your body when you eat sugar, you are also causing a degree of metabolic and physiological mayhem.

Until about 100 years ago, the average annual intake of sugar in Western countries was about 20 pounds per person. Even this was part of a diet that included far more "natural" vitamin- and mineral-rich foods than is currently the case. The present annual intake of sugar in the US is over 100 pounds per person. The human body is very adaptable, but it takes more than a century to get used to such a change in nutritional intake.

Organs such as the pancreas (the source of insulin and essential protein-digesting enzymes) are grossly overworked when sugar plays a large part in the diet. The pancreas, when faced with sugar, pumps out insulin. This has the job of maintaining the proper level of sugar in the bloodstream. Insulin is also released in response to stimulant drinks, such as coffee and tea, which initially cause (as does stress) a release by the liver of stored sugar. Thus a diet rich in sugar, and which contains the usual amount of tea, coffee and alcohol (as well as cola drinks and chocolates, which also contain caffeine) will produce a situation in which a major organ is grossly overworked. With this sort of pattern, the fluctuations in blood sugar levels, boosted by dietary and liver-stored sugar and then depressed and controlled by the pancreatic insulin, have a profound effect upon the health and personality of the individual. At the same time, because of the sugar-rich diet, it is less likely that people will eat enough of the foods containing vitamins and minerals to allow them to meet the minimum standards of nutrition. Thus, other systems in the body become deficient, including the immune system. This whole process may of course take years, all the while accompanied by declining well-being and an unnoticed rise in Candida activity. Sugar has been well described as pure, white, and deadly.

For the first few weeks of the program (three weeks to be safe), even fresh fruit should be avoided because of its high content of natural fruit sugars. Even when fruit consumption is resumed after the three-week break, it should not include very sweet melons, which are too high in sugar for the Candida sufferer (and often contain mold).

Milk contains its own form of sugar, and this is also considered undesirable throughout the program. Pasteurized milk encourages Candida.[9] The exception to this is yogurt—if it is natural and "live," which will be clearly stated on its container. There are many "dead" yogurts and a good many have sugar addded. These are completely unsuitable to the program. Live yogurt itself is helpful because it contains bacteria that inhibit Candida and that assist (along with acidophilus, which is often used in yogurt culture) in the repopulation of the bowel by beneficial microorganisms.

Other Foods to Avoid

It is best to avoid smoked meats and fish, sausages, corned beef, hot dogs, and hamburgers because of the substances added to them, some of which derive from yeasts. Nuts, other than freshly cracked ones, should also be avoided, because they attract mold as they become rancid. Any foods that have been kept for a while, other than in a frozen state, are liable to be slightly moldy, and these should be avoided too.

You now have a picture of the type of foods not to eat: mainly the yeast- and fungus-related foods, as well as the refined carbohydrates and anything containing them.

Your adherence to such a program may depend upon many things, but none more than motivation. Just how much do you want to get better, and how much effort are you prepared to make? It is really not up to anyone but you. Certainly, taking supplements as described, will go a long way toward that end. So will avoiding yeasts and foods derived from them. But by putting the whole program together, including the sugar-free aspect of the diet, you really give the system a chance to work quickly and work well.

What you can still eat is varied and interesting. Below, I have outlined a diet that is nutritious, tasty, and above all, anti-Candida.

Once you have followed this pattern for a while, it is unlikely that you will ever really want to reintroduce most of the "undesirables," even when Candida is back under control.

Dietary Pattern

It is suggested that three meals be eaten daily, and that meals not be skipped unless you are off-color and really have no appetite.

Breakfasts

A high-fiber diet is best suited to defeating Candida. In Professor Jeffrey Bland's words, "The diet should be higher than normal in fiber, using oat bran fiber to increase the absorptive surface of the fecal material and also hasten the elimination of metabolic by-products."[16] Choose therefore from the following, for a wholesome and non-Candida-supporting breakfast.

1. Cooked oatmeal. Add a little cinnamon and some ground cashews for additional flavor. Use no sugar or honey. Make with water, not milk.
2. Mixed seed and nut breakfast (combine sunflower, pumpkin, sesame, and linseed together with oatmeal or flaked millet). These can be eaten as they are, or soaked overnight in a little water to make a softer texture, or moistened with natural live yogurt. Add wheat germ and freshly ground nuts if desired.
3. Alternate days: two eggs, any style except raw.
4. Bread or toast (made without yeast or sugar) and butter.

5. Brown rice kedgeree (rice and fish).
6. Whole wheat or rice and oat pancakes (no sweetening).
7. Natural live yogurt (add wheat germ if desired).
8. After the first week or so of the program, fresh fruit can be added to the menu; for example, item 1 or 2 could be complemented by sliced banana or grated apple or item 7 could have fresh fruit added, or fruit could be eaten as a major part of the meal, with a handful of fresh nuts and/or seeds, such as sunflower, pumpkin, and so on.
9. Fish (not smoked) or meat (not cured or salted).
10. Whole wheat or whole rice, and yogurt (ensure no sugar in cereals). The use of muesli-type breakfast mixtures is in order if they are homemade. If commercially prepared, they will contain dried fruit and nuts of almost certain rancidity, and frequently sugar or honey as well.

By the simple mixing of oat flakes or millet flakes with fresh nuts or seeds, as mentioned in items 1 and 2 above, it is possible to have a high-fiber, nutritious, and tasty meal. If selections from 1 and 2 are eaten, then a high fiber content will be ensured, so these are suggested as the most desirable. If any of the other choices are eaten, add a heaping teaspoon of a 50-50 mixture of linseed and bran to the meal or swallow at the end of the meal with a little water.

Remember to chew all food, especially carbohydrates, thoroughly. There is no way in which half-chewed carbohydrates can be digested, because the enzymes present in saliva are essential to the breakdown of these foods. For this reason, it is undesirable to drink with meals, as the liquid is frequently used as a moistening agent to facilitate swallowing, which as a result reduces efficient chewing. A high fiber meal is not only ideal for providing the type of food needed for the anti-Candida program, it also ensures a steady release of natural sugars into the blood stream, rather than the immediate rise produced by refined sugar-rich foods. Fiber helps keep blood-sugar levels even, avoiding ups and downs in energy and mood, which can trigger the craving for a quick "sugar fix."

Drinks at breakfast time should consist of either green tea, China tea, herb tea (such as camomile), all unsweetened; or a mineral water, such as Perrier.

Main Meals

You should have no great problem in finding appealing food during the strict avoidance period of the diet. The one area of contention exists in the choice of animal proteins. Most commercial meat and poultry contains residues of the antibiotics and hormonal substances that are fed to the animals in the process of raising them for market. This means that regular eating of beef, pork, or chicken, unless it is from a source known to avoid such methods, is a potential danger to the success of the whole program (and a health hazard at all times). Indeed, it is probable that this factor is a major, yet unrecognized, element in the whole Candida scenario. While the use of antibiotics and steroids in medications can be relatively easily remembered and identified in your personal medical history, it is impossible to know just how much of these same substances you have ingested on a daily basis through food.

For this reason it is suggested that efforts be made to track down non-steroid-fed meat and poultry, in which antibiotics have not been used. In major cities this is probably possible. In California, for example, there is a chain of supermarkets (Mrs. Gooch's Ranch Markets) that provides a complete range of meats and poultry that is guaranteed free of all contamination. Lamb and mutton are less likely to be affected by additives, as are rabbit and any other game meat, or poultry. Fish is safe, apart from other sources of pollution, which do not concern Candida directly. For the duration of the diet, therefore, it is suggested that unless meat or poultry can be definitely identified as free of hormones or antibiotics, meat should be limited to game, rabbit (unless farmed), mutton, or lamb. Fish, of course, can be eaten regularly as well.

Ideally, in order to maintain the high-fiber diet that is so desirable when Candida is active, the two main meals of the day should include as many fresh vegetables as possible. These should be eaten both raw and cooked, and an excellent pattern to adopt is as follows. One of the main meals each day should be source of protein, such as fish, poultry, lamb, egg, or fresh nuts, together with as large a mixed salad as imagination can conjure and appetite permits. The other main meal should also contain protein, in addition to cooked vegetables. The source of protein at each meal does not, of course, have to be based on animals. The combining of a grain and legumes (brown rice and lentils, or millet and chickpeas) at the same meal ensures adequate protein.

What is essential is that adequate protein be eaten daily, whether from a "safe" animal source, or from the proper combining of complementary vegetable proteins. An adequate amount for one person, however, may not necessarily be so for another. For example, as a rule, Asians require, for good health, less protein than people from northern Europe. The difference lies in the efficiency with which Asians digest and absorb the protein they do eat. Thus 50 g a day of high-quality protein is adequate for an Asian, and 75 g (or more depending upon activity) may be required by a Caucasian.[5]

Since natural, live yogurt (a source of protein) is going to play a part in the anti-Candida diet, it is unlikely that eating protein at both of the main meals, in addition to this, is necessary. It should be possible to have, for example, a mixed salad, with a baked potato or savory rice dish and additional nuts and seeds for one meal, while having a "safe" animal protein and a variety of cooked vegetables at the other. In any case, individual tastes and preferences will differ markedly, and the variations available are so great that no more than broad guidelines need be given. The essentials are to ensure the following:

• Avoid all yeast-based, or yeast-containing, foods.

- Avoid all sugar and refined grain products, and foods containing them.
- Avoid all fermented foods and drinks.
- Avoid meats containing residues of antibiotics and steroids.
- Do eat three meals daily.
- Do ensure adequate protein intake.
- Do ensure that a high fiber content is maintained.
- Avoid fruit for the first three or four weeks of the program.

Once symptoms begin to abate, and you find that you would like to increase the range of foods slightly, it is, of course, permissible to experiment a bit. This should not be before the end of the second month on the program, and then only if there has been a marked improvement. When you introduce a food that has been on the "avoid" list, observe the consequences carefully. If there are none, you might extend your experiment to another food after a week or so. If symptoms return, go back to basic avoidance, as specified above, until they calm down again. I am not saying that you *must* experiment in this way, only that if you do, or if you feel constrained by the limitations imposed by the program, then at least do it carefully, with the knowledge that it might (only might) upset things. If it does, it just means being patient for a little longer. There are many excellent books available that explain the principles of rotation diets and that can help in formulating a strategy for eating certain foods only periodically but in a systematic way.[28] It is not suggested that the reintroduction of foods containing sugar be started at this stage, other than in a very minimal sense, perhaps introducing something like pasta or honey.

Other Essential Information Regarding Food

Molds are present on most fruits and vegetables, so these should be washed well and eaten fresh, for obviously the longer they are kept, the more the mold will develop.

Steaming vegetables is the best way to retain the vital minerals so often destroyed and lost in boiling. Dressing a salad with lemon juice, olive oil, and a little natural yogurt can replace the vinegar or other dressings not compatible with the program.

Yeasts also grow on grains of all sorts, so the fresher these are the better. Many people with Candida problems are allergic to grains. This allergy may well diminish during the program of Candida control, and a little experimentation is in order after two or three months if symptoms generally have declined.

A reminder regarding nuts: peanuts and pistachios, in particular, are subject to mold (in the case of peanuts, this mold is a highly toxic, potentially cancer-causing agent). All nuts, unless freshly cracked by you, will contain some degree of mold, and certainly a degree of rancidity of the natural oils. Eat current-season nuts, freshly cracked by yourself, or else avoid them.

Apart from a little butter and natural, live yogurt, avoid all milk products (Truss does allow cottage cheese).

If you are forced to eat at a restaurant or if friends invite you for a meal, make sure that you stick to basics. Avoid sauces and gravy; avoid desserts; avoid stuffing or any obvious undesirables, such as mushrooms. A meat, poultry, or fish dish, with salad or vegetables, is the safest bet, and stick to water instead of wine.

What about sugar substitutes for those who cannot keep away from sweet things? These are open to question as far as long-term safety is concerned, but in small amounts, for the duration of the program (at least six months) they at least do not encourage Candida. Aspartame and saccharin fall into this category, but not fructose, corn syrup, or any other sugar-rich substitute for the real thing.

Remember that all commercial breakfast foods, such as corn flakes, are undesirable. They are processed, and most contain yeast and/or sugar products.

Water from the tap should be filtered before drinking if possible.

There are many inexpensive water filters available, and filtering will remove a variety of organic substances that otherwise would find their way into food, or directly into you. Most bottled water is acceptable, but ensure it is not carbonated if you have problems with bloating and gas. As for coffee and tea, they are a sticking point for many. They are undesirable, not only as sources of mold, but because they stimulate sugar release from the liver. This sugar stimulates pancreatic activity, which exhausts this vital organ further, and feeds the Candida. There are other good reasons for not using tea, as it reduces the efficiency of both protein and iron absorption by the body; and coffee is suspected of involvement in certain forms of cancer. Herb teas are often better, and some have been found to help in the control of Candida, and related problems (Rooibos, a South African tea, used as a tea substitute, and by allergic people) and taheebo (helpful in catarrhal problems) are worth trying if you can find them (try a health food store).

As the program produces results, and symptoms become tolerable or disappear, you can reintroduce a limited quantity of foods based on, or containing, mold or yeast. Wine or real ale in limited amounts, or tea, may be taken occasionally. However, the need for vigilance continues, because it is not the aim of the program to remove Candida from the scene altogether, nor would this be possible. Even if the problem is attacked vigorously with the use of antifungal drugs as well as the program outlined above, the yeast will remain in the body.

The long-term answer, after initially controlling the yeast by these means, is to maintain a high level of immune function, by respect for what the diet should contain, in terms of nutritional value, as well as avoidance of those factors that you know can reduce its ability to defend you. This does not mean that the program is a life sentence. Hope that after a while, you will no longer crave sweets, or even enjoy sweet foods. Also hope that your new sense of well-being will motivate you toward following the pattern of eating suggested permanently, because you actually enjoy it as well as because it is good for you.

Other Factors

Not only is it important to avoid foods and beverages containing fungal or yeast substances, but also to avoid inhaling these organisms or their spores. This is the reason for keeping away from damp, dank places and for dealing with the presence of any mold and wet or dry rot that might be present in your environment. If there is any danger of dampness in rooms, cupboards, cellars, or lofts, do something positive about dealing with "this," or, if absolutely necessary, move to a new, dry place of residence. *Your home might be making you ill.* This advice especially applies to anyone who notices a worsening of symptoms in damp or muggy weather, or who is obviously affected by contact with moldy or dank environments.

Full-spectrum light is another important element that can improve immune and general function.[29] It is known that the eyes contain photo receptors that carry impulses directly to the pituitary gland. This is the "master" gland of the body and is vital to normal health and function. If the eyes are denied light (not artificial light, but the full spectrum from the sun), then demonstrable imbalances occur in the hormonal system as a direct result. Behavioral and physical symptoms can occur. The immune system is also affected, and this is the reason for our interest. The advice to all who wear glasses, or who spend most of their days indoors behind glass, is that they should get outside for at least half an hour a day, with nothing between natural light and their eyes. If going out is not possible, then spend the time by an open window, without glasses or contact lenses. In a polluted city, the light getting through is distorted to a degree, and so more exposure is required. This does not mean looking at the sun, even on an overcast day; just being outdoors is enough if the eyes are not shielded.

Full-spectrum fluorescent lighting units are now available. It has been found that health and productivity improve dramatically when such lighting is introduced into the workplace. As one of the additional supports for the immune system, access to unpolluted, unfiltered, pure light is a positive step.

The immune system also benefits from adequate exercise. This means trying to apply the ideals set out in Dr. Kenneth Cooper's book *Aerobics*.[30] At least every other day, you should participate in a form of physical exercise sufficient to stimulate the circulation and respiration. A brisk walk of one or two miles is the safest and easiest form of exercise that can produce such results. The book mentioned should be read, and its graded advice followed. Its beauty lies in that it applies to anyone, at any stage of fitness, so that readers can gradually lift themselves to their own level of optimum fitness.

Reducing stress and anxiety is fundamental to health, as is our requirement for TLC (tender loving care). Many popular and readily available books emphasize emotional and spiritual well-being. The study of relaxation, meditation, and general stress-reducing methods benefits the immune system. I have outlined a program of stress reduction in my book on the subject,[31] to help in both assessing and dealing with those stress factors that affect life.

In considering the overall importance of the immune system, it is worth commenting on an area of medical research that tends to be ignored, because of its unpopular message. There is abundant proof that women who are promiscuous, or who are sexually involved with several men, are more prone to cancer of the womb than those who are sexually involved with only one or a few partners.[5] Early sexual experience is also shown to predispose a person toward diseases that should be prevented by an intact immune system. AIDS is more common among homosexuals who have multiple partners, than among those who have steady relationships with a single partner. It would seem, therefore, that close physical contact of a sexual nature plays a role in the functioning of the immune system. It is assumed that calling on the immune system to cope with antigens from a wide variety of different sources (remember that sperm is a foreign protein to the body) could well be a factor in depleting the immune response of an individual (along with a great number of other factors).

This viewpoint has been expressed in numerous medical journals since the AIDS epidemic began.[32] It points to a necessary return to relative fidelity, in sexual terms, for anyone who wishes to maintain an intact immune system. This does not mean that celibacy is called for, but that frequent changes in sexual partners are to be avoided. This is desirable in both heterosexual and homosexual relationships, at least during the program against Candida.

In the next chapter, we will briefly consider other methods by which some practitioners attempt to control Candida.

Note: It should be clear from the discussions in this chapter that there should be no intake of antibiotics, steroids, or the contraceptive pill during the course of the anti-Candida program unless absolutely vital.

6

Additional Methods of Candida Control

By relying on diet and supplementation it is not only possible to control Candida, but to improve general well-being dramatically. This is something no medication can achieve, no matter how few side effects it produces. However, we will take a look at some of the medications used to help control Candida, as well as two other methods, so that our discussion of control methods is complete.

Nystatin

The treatment of a fungal infection, such as Candida, by medication, involves the use of antifungal antibiotics, such as nystatin. This is active against a wide range of yeasts and yeast-like fungi, including Candida. This drug comes in a variety of forms: as a liquid, for use in the mouth; as tablets, for use in treating Candida in the intestinal tract; as suppositories, for use in the vagina; and as creams, ointments, and powders, for the treatment of surface areas, nails, and so on.

Nystatin is lethal to yeast cells on contact. Getting it into contact with them is not always easy, especially if the area involved is deep in the bowel. The nystatin, passing through, will kill surface yeasts, but any that are imbedded deeper into the wall of the intestine will remain untouched. Absorption of nystatin is poor, so little reaches the bloodstream.

There is general consensus that nystatin is well tolerated and causes few side effects.[2, 9] The major reason for not using it is that it deals only with the short-term situation. If a condition such as Candida has become so widespread as to cause a problem, then it is vital that the immune system and bowel flora, which should be controlling the situation, are revitalized. Reliance on nystatin will leave the immune system in the same state, except that over time, there will be fewer yeast by-products entering the bloodstream to challenge the immune system. This, it is thought (by Truss, Crook, and others), allows the immune system to revive gradually. There is certainly no objection to nystatin being used if the condition is severe enough to warrant it, but this should be done in combination with the program outlined in the previous chapters. Otherwise, there will be only short-term gains and the condition will recur. Nystatin is itself derived from a mold source and can cause allergic symptoms in sensitive individuals. Some patients become dependent on nystatin and have difficulty weaning themselves from it.

The dosage of nystatin is usually about 2 million units daily (four tablets of half a million units each), but double this dosage is relatively safe. Side effects are limited to nausea, vomiting, and diarrhea, which occur only with very high doses (over 4 million units daily).

The above information should not be taken as an explicit recommendation for the use of nystatin. The major recommendations given in this book regarding the control of Candida by natural rather than medicinal methods are effective in the majority of cases. Taking nystatin does not necessarily shorten the process of control, and indeed may result in the individual relying on medication, thus allowing the supporting anti-Candida program to lapse.

Copper Aspirinate

Dr. Bland has discussed the use of a combination of the mineral copper with aspirin, in the form of a copper aspirinate compound, in the treatment of Candida. This, he points out,[16] provides in one tablet 10 mg of copper daily and 330 mg of aspirin. This apparently reduces the symptoms of Candida infection associated with intestinal irritation and inflammation. He describes the research of Dr. J. Sorenson, who has called this preparation "one of the most powerful anti-inflammatory substances studied to date."[33] It has both an anti-inflammatory and an anti-fungal role to play, according to this research.

As far as the use of copper aspirinate in the anti-Candida program is concerned, it must be clear that while being of possible short-term use, it does not comply with the description "natural," in that a pharmaceutical drug effect is clearly being aimed at, rather than the bolstering of the defense mechanism, or a biological attack upon Candida, such as that foreseen when using acidophilus. This does not mean that copper aspirinate should not be used, only that it is not part of the program recommended in this book. Its limited availability is another reason for not regarding it at least as an alternative in the opening phases of the program. Bland suggests its use, especially in cases in which intestinal factors play a large part in the symptom picture, for the first two to three weeks of the program.

Caprystatin

The anti-fungal activity of certain fatty acids has been demonstrated by investigators such as Neuhauser,[40] who has shown that dilute (0.01) caprylic acid (coconut extract) destroys Candida effectively. He has successfully treated patients with severe intestinal Candida by using caprylic acid in a form that allows a timed release as it passes through the bowel. If not in a timed-release form, the caprylic acid is ineffective, being absorbed in the upper intestinal region. Caprylic acid mimics the fatty acids produced by normal bowel flora, which are a major factor in the body's control over Candida. (see "Further Information" for the manufacturer's address.)

Colonics and Enemas

Colonic irrigation involves the administration of water, sometimes combined with other substances, into the bowel in order to clear debris from the region and to promote its health. Useful in this respect are garlic extract, oxygen, and acidophilus (or as Crook suggests, nystatin). By making repeated applications of water, coupled with one of these additives, there is every chance of greatly influencing the condition of the bowel. Enemas are less effective, since they penetrate only a short distance, unlike the colonic irrigation, which can pass water the length of the large bowel. The technique requires expert skills, and its use in Candida problems would require additional knowledge. In principle, however, such treatment is recommended, at least in the early stages of the program. There is no reason why acidophilus should not be administered in this way, rather than just orally, to assist in the repopulation of beneficial flora in the bowel and the control of Candida.

Desensitization

Carefully controlled doses of Candida extract may be injected in the hope of producing a response from the immune system. Antibodies thus produced by white blood cells are useful in assisting the defense against antigens entering the system because of the yeast. The use of yeast extracts as a "vaccine" also appears to assist general immune function, by helping to balance or regulate aspects of the system relating to "helper" and "suppressor" cells, as discussed in Chapter 2, "Candida and your Defense System."

The whole exercise is complicated in the extreme, because while Candida albicans is a strain of yeast that is clearly identifiable, it contains within its make-up a large number of variables. Thus the Candida that is growing in one person is not exactly the same as that growing in another. This biological individuality applies to yeasts just as much as to every other living creature, including people.

Thus, the same extract of Candida, injected into two people, will not produce the same results. Not only is the yeast likely to prove different from the one to which the person is usually exposed, but his/her individuality requires a process of trial and error, in order to find and fight the particular strain of Candida present in his/her system. Heredity may be largely responsible for the different responses of individuals to such treatment. The practitioner who is employing anti-Candida desensitization treatment must be an expert in the field and understand the complex variables.

Even should such expertise be available, this approach, with all its possible pitfalls in terms of variable reactions, can at best deal with only one aspect of the problem. It may assist in bolstering the immune system against the by-products of Candida's infestation. This is especially desirable for those people who are suffering from certain allergy symptoms mentioned earlier. But it will do little for the local symptoms currently active in the bowel or reproductive system. Only those harmful effects that are countered by the bloodstream will be affected. Valuable as this may be, it would leave much of the underlying condition the same, and would still call for the program of anti-Candida diet and supplements in order to control its spread and deny it its nutrients.

Truss points out that the use of this type of "vaccination" program is not recommended for patients suffering from auto-immune conditions. These include rheumatoid arthritis. Stimulation of the immune response in someone who is being attacked by his own immune system would aggravate the condition.

Truss has written:

> I obtain yeast from supply houses that have been made aware of the necessity of bio-assaying each new batch on humans. Prior to their being informed of this fact, they were putting out a number of batches that would not give a positive skin test on known reactors. The preparation as I order it, is simply Candida albicans 1:10.[34]

This indicates one more difficulty in this method: it is vital that the

Candida extract used is actually active, and that this be proved in each batch produced; otherwise the pitfalls described above are compounded.

These last two anti-Candida methods are the major forms of treatment recommended by both Truss and Crook. They do, of course, strongly advocate the natural, dietary approach, especially to prevent Candida from spreading, as well as to support other treatments.

The following case histories will give an indication of the way in which the "natural" approach works.

7

Case Histories

Mr. E. M., age 36

This young man, employed as a local government officer, consulted me in 1982, for seven years, his health had been declining dramatically. His major symptoms included bloating of the abdomen, accompanied by nausea and flatulence, heartburn, and indigestion. Constipation had become chronic. There was a tendency to light headedness and dizziness. He had periodic attacks of shivering, followed by high temperature, which incapacitated him.

The onset of the condition, previous to which his health was unremarkable, came after an attack of gastroenteritis while on vacation. Treatment had, naturally enough, been with a broad-spectrum antibiotic. In his own words:

> For the eighteen months following [the gastroenteritis] I suffered all
> the symptoms daily. They were so severe, they resulted in my being
> unable to work for six months, and the remaining twelve months
> I was able to work only because I had support from my colleagues,
> who shared my work load, and understanding superiors, who allowed
> me to go home, or rest, when the attacks were extremely severe.

There had been a gradual improvement over the following years until some twelve months prior to my seeing him, when, after an acute attack, he was left with all the symptoms described above. At that time he wrote, "At present I am struggling to cope with each day as it comes, and deal with this extremely debilitating and distressing illness as best I can."

In the years between the onset of his illness and consulting me, he had been seen by numerous doctors. An endoscopy showed no disease of the bowel. He was checked for what is called a mal-absorption problem, and again no abnormality was discerned. He went to a homeopathic hospital on two occasions, and consulted an herbalist, an osteopath and an allergy specialist (a clinical ecologist). He was placed on a rotation diet, which helped him to avoid repetitive contact with suspected food families, but which had little effect on his condition.

When I first saw him, his diet was as follows: Breakfast con-sisted of *bacon* and tomato or *sausages*, *rice cakes* and *marmalade*. Decaffeinated *coffee* and *fruit juice* (not freshly squeezed). Mid-morning he had fresh fruit. Lunch was a salad and a baked potato plus *ham* or cottage cheese. The evening meal was either *chicken*, or *pork*, or *sausages*, or fish and vegetables. He had *rice cakes* and a hot *milk* drink before retiring. I have italicized those foods that are avoided in the anti-Candida diet.

He appeared exhausted, but was a bright and intelligent patient who I felt would cooperate actively in any program designed to assist recovery.

After tests, including cytotoxic tests to identify specific foods to which he might be reacting, as well as hair analysis (low in chromium, iron, manganese and selenium), he was prescribed the following:

- An anti-yeast, anti fungal diet low in carbohydrates.
- Supplements of vitamins A, E, B_1, B_2, B_3, B_6, calcium panto-thenate (B_5), calcium, magnesium, and manganese. Vitamin C was also added. The vitamin A was in emulsified form for easy absorption.
- The pattern of eating was to include a seed and yogurt breakfast, a salad lunch, and an evening meal of "safe" protein with vegetables.

At that time information about biotin and acidophilus was not at hand, and the above program, which the reader will recognize as a modified version of that given in earlier chapters, had a remarkable effect. Improvement began soon after he began the program. Two months later, biotin and acidophilus were introduced. Six months after the first visit, he reported at least a 50 percent improvement in all symptoms; there were still some days of exhaustion, but overall an upward trend in health was noted after seven years of decline.

Confirmation of the involvement of Candida came with an attempt, early in the program, to introduce an organic iron supplement, in a liquid yeast-based form. This was met with an immediate return of constipation, which had nearly resolved itself. A check up six months later found continued improvement, with lapses in the diet producing confirmatory flare-ups. There is no reason to doubt that the condition will be kept under control, and that the health of the patient will continue to improve. A letter just eighteen months after the start of the program states, "Please accept apologies for delay in contacting you. It is an indication of the progress we have made that I am well enough not to have to adhere so strictly. I am very much better overall." (Letter dated November 8, 1984.)

Mrs. E. V., age 50

This patient consulted me with a history of extreme itching and inflammation of the skin of the neck and scalp, of one year's duration. She had an earlier history of acne, which was treated by antibiotic therapy (unsuccessfully). She suffered from flatulence and had a history of colitis and a "delicate" digestive system. She had consulted an herbalist with little result, and a hypnotist who taught her relaxation and helped her to stop scratching the area. The condition remained as before.

At the time of the consultation, I was not yet aware of the work of Truss on Candida and my approach was to use a nutritional supplement, based on her general clinical picture, a nutrition questionnaire, a hair analysis, and her current symptoms. Her diet was excellent (which, because this turned out to be a Candida problem, had probably saved her from far wider infestation). She was placed on the following supplements, each taken daily: emulsified vitamin A, 60,000 IU.; zinc orotate, 200 mg; calcium and magnesium orotates, 1 g each; chromium orotate, 10 mg; selenium, 50 mcg; and oil of evening primrose (vitamin F), 1 g. I also suggested that she take yeast tablets as a source of vitamin B. At this point she wrote to me (she lived a considerable distance from my practice) saying, "I am following your suggestions carefully, except for the brewer's yeast. Over the years I have tried a number of times to take it, but it creates gas and is most unpleasant."

This set off alarm bells, for I had just read the first of Truss's articles that week. I immediately revised her diet, which, while good under usual conditions, contained substances derived from yeast, and of course a certain amount of "yeast food" such as honey and muesli bars. The patient canceled her following appointment with the comment that, as her symptoms had disappeared, she felt the journey unnecessary. I quite agreed. A year later she remained symptom-free, including both skin and bowel conditions.

Mrs. D. B., age 31

I was consulted by this lady, a computer programmer, with the following list of complaints: eyes bloodshot and irritated for the past nine months; odd aches, in joints and muscles; fingers slightly swollen, puffiness under eyes (and sometimes above) after sleep. Ten years after the onset of her symptoms she had had cosmetic surgery and had taken diuretics, to no avail. She had been on a macrobiotic diet, with no improvement. Her periods were erratic and painful, and her breasts swelled and became sensitive at period time. She felt unnaturally tired much of the time, and there was a family history of bronchial problems and depression, from which she, too, suffered.

Her current diet was as follows: Breakfast: consisted of commercially prepared *muesli* with *added sugar* plus *milk* or apple juice (once a week she had eggs, *bacon,* and *sausage* for breakfast). Lunch was cooked vegetables or *sandwiches.* The Evening meal was fish and rice, and occasionally meat. During the day she has something *sweet*, three cups of *tea* with *sugar*, and *cookies*. She had noticed a progressive inability to cope with alcohol.

Her diet was reformed to remove the sugars and milk, and to increase complex carbohydrates. She was prescribed (after appropriate tests) vitamin B-complex, kelp, oil of evening primrose, vitamin B_2, glutamic acid (an amino acid), and the minerals chromium, iron, manganese, and selenium. Also prescribed were biotin and acidophilus, after meals. Within two months, she reported that her period was regular for the first time in years, there had been a less overall tendency to swell (eyes or breasts), and she was able to handle alcohol. (It was, in fact, proscribed from her diet, which raises the problem of patients complying with instructions—a major headache for practitioners.) Three months later her condition was vastly improved, and her tiredness, bloodshot eyes, and aches in muscles and joints had all diminished to a point where they no longer bothered her. A year later she was symptom free.

Miss G. H., age 29

The tragic progression of ill health in this case is a clear indictment of the failure of many health professionals to recognize Candida when it is staring them in the face.

Before consulting me, this woman wrote to me as follows:

> I have been suffering from pelvic inflammatory disease (PID) for almost two years now. The problem started when I began to experience lower abdominal pain and feel generally unwell. I was, at the time, using the contraceptive IUD, which I had removed, believing this to be the cause of the pain. [Prior to this, it turned out, the young woman

had been using the contraceptive pill, and had a history of recurrent thrush.] However, this [removal of the IUD] had no effect and the pain became worse. Unfortunately my GP [general practitioner—her family doctor] did not diagnose PID, and I therefore received no treatment in the early stages of the disease. Eventually I went to the hospital, where the gynecologist diagnosed PID by means of a laparoscopy. At that time there was some damage to the fallopian tubes and adhesions in the pelvic area. I was put on antibiotics, and for a time the condition seemed to improve. After a short time, however, I began to experience further attacks, and had to take larger doses of antibiotics regularly, and strong pain-killers for much of the time. At times the pain was incredibly intense. In January, 1983, I was admitted to a women's hospital in London for another laparoscopy. They found that both fallopian tubes were blocked, and it sounded as though damage/adhesions in the pelvic area had progressed. Despite this I was told that the pain I was complaining of was psychological, and though they would be prepared to do tube reconstruction for fertility purposes, there was nothing more they could do for me.

I visited a specialist in February, 1983, who said that my symptoms and pain were classic PID, but there was nothing he could do to help....

My menstrual cycle had now gone from four to six weeks. Apart from the pain, other symptoms were active nausea, stomach upset, dizziness, and slightly raised temperature. I also became very depressed. In July, 1983, I had surgery after consulting a leading gynecologist at Hammersmith Hospital. This consisted of removal of the left fallopian tube and reconstruction of the right; separation of adhesions to the tubes, ovaries, and uterus through microsurgery; presacral neurotomy [removal of the nerve to the uterus]; and steroid treatment to prevent regrowth of adhesions.

After this, all was well until early November, 1983, when symptoms began again. Although the pain was not as severe, tests showed the infection was active again. I was put on heavy doses of antibiotics. It did not clear up, and I am now in my sixth week of antibiotics. The specialist told me that there was nothing more they can do surgically, and that I may have the condition for the rest of my life, and must learn to live with it. I have a very positive attitude towards getting better, and find it very difficult to believe that there is nothing else I can do to beat this disease, or at least fight it more effectively.

The patient's history indicated that she had commenced on this sad slide to ill health at the age of twelve, when cystitis was first apparent, after which she soon began a thirteen-year history of vaginal thrush.

In late January, 1984, this patient was placed on the program outlined in earlier chapters: high fiber, low refined carbohydrate; no fungal foods; and supplements of biotin, acidophilus, olive oil, zinc, vitamin F, and garlic. Two months later, she reported that she was feeling much better, apart from a couple of bad spells from which she recovered more quickly than usual.

A letter dated January 10, 1985, reads as follows, "I have been feeling considerably better. The pain problem is now limited to a few days a month (around period time). After my last laparoscopy, the specialist said that it was the best result from that type of operation that he'd ever had. My remaining fallopian tube was tested and is clear, so I am a lot happier in myself." This is a clear and dramatic example of the tragedy that occurs when Candida becomes active in a young body, and of the effectiveness of the program outlined in this book.

Miss S. R., age 35

This young actress suffered from continuous facial acne, which was both unsightly and a disadvantage in her work, as well as being psychologically upsetting. This condition has been present since the age of fourteen. Her past history was unremarkable, apart from a highly stressful lifestyle, surgical intervention (cryo-surgery) to deal with a cervical erosion, and a tendency not to ovulate regularly. When under stress in the past, her skin erupted into very large pustules. By following the anti-Candida program (as outlined in earlier chapters) her skin was normal and she was ovulating regularly after only three months. Improvement has been maintained for the past year.

Candida is possibly the least understood and most widespread cause of ill health currently in our midst. Precisely because it is known to be everywhere, it is largely ignored, and not even considered in the diagnosis of conditions such as PID. The cases quoted by Truss, which include cases similar to those I have described here, as well as individuals who were diagnosed as having schizophrenia, manic depression, and multiple sclerosis, deserve attention. All of these pathological conditions were restored to normality with the nutritional program we have been considering, together with anti-yeast medication.

Greater awareness of this diagnosis as a possibility would, perhaps, lead to a marked reduction in human suffering. Candida is not just a minor health irritant. It can destroy the physical and mental cohesion of the individual in a very short time. Prevention is practiced by the same means as those described for treatment. The knowledge that we now have about controlling Candida is easy to understand and easily put to practical use.

Self-help is always necessary. It can take 50 years, or more, for the penetration of an idea to permeate the medical profession as a whole. Let us hope that with modern communication and the help of the media, this process will be speeded up in the case of Candida. The name of Dr. C. Orion Truss, of Birmingham, Alabama, will eventually become well known throughout medicine. He deserves the gratitude of us all for his research into Candida albicans and its role in much ill health.

FURTHER INFORMATION

Supplement Supplies

Supplements can be obtained from health food stores, or from the following suppliers:

Freeda Vitamins
36 East 41st Street
New York, NY 10017
Tel: 212-685-4980
(source of yeast-free supplements, caprystatin, and Vital Dophilus)

Arteria
1061-B Shary Circle
Concord, CA 94518
Tel: 415-827-2636
(source of caprystatin)

Natren, Inc.
10935 Camarillo Street
North Hollywood, CA 91602
(source of Megadophilus)

Recommended Reading

C. Orion Truss, MD, *The Missing Diagnosis,* obtainable from author,
   PO Box 26508, Birmingham, Alabama 35226.

William G. Crook, MD, *The Yeast Connection,* obtainable from author,
   PO Box 3494, Jackson, Tennessee 38301.

Journal of Alternative Medicine, obtainable from 30 Station Approach,
   West Byfleet, Surrey, England.

REFERENCES

1. Roger Williams, *Biochemical Individuality* (University of Texas Press, 1979).

2. C. Orion Truss, MD, *Missing Diagnosis* (see Further Information for address).

3. Jay Stein (ed.), *Internal Medicine* (Little Brown, 1983.)

4. R. Williams and G. Deason, *Proceedings of National Academy of Sciences* (USA, 57, p. 1638, 1968).

5. Jeffrey Bland, PhD, *Medical Applications of Clinical Nutrition* (Keats, 1983).

6. Jeffrey Bland, PhD, *Nutraerobics* (Harper & Row, 1983).

7. Dr. Michael Colgan, *Your Personal Vitamin Profile* (Blond & Briggs, 1983).

8. Roger Williams, PhD, *Nutrition against Disease* (Bantam, 1981).

9. W.M. Crook, MD, *The Yeast Connection* (Professional Books, 1984).

10. *Journal of Orthomolecular Psychiatry,* Vol. 9, No. 4 (1980), pp. 287-301

11. W. Philpott and D. Kalita, *Brain Allergies* (Keats, 1980).

12. Dr. W. Hemmings, *Food Antigens in the Gut* (Lancaster Press, 1980).

13. K. Shahani and A. Ayeno, "Role of dietary lactobacilli in gastrointestinal microecology," *American Journal of Clinical Nutrition,* Vol. 33 (Nov. 1980), pp. 2448-57.

14. M. Speck, "Contributions of micro organisms to foods and nutrition," *Nutrition News,* Vol. 38, No. 4 (1975), 13.

15. G. Reddy et al., "Natural antibiotic activity of Lactobacillus acidophilus and bulgaricus," *Cultured Dairy Products Journal,* Vol. 18, No. 2 (1983), p. 15.

16. Dr. Jeffrey Bland, PhD, "Candida Albicans—An alternative therapy for an unexpected problem," *Journal of Alternative Medicine,* July 1983, pp. 18-19.

17. *Medical Science Proceedings* (Yamaguchi, 1982).

18. *Applied Microbiology* June 1969; Lloyd Harris, *The Book of Garlic* (Aris Books, 1979).

19. *Medical Journal of Australia,* Vol. 1, No. 60 (1982).

20. Tyarcke and Gos, "Inhibitory action of garlic on growth and respiration of micro organisms" (1979).

21. *Mycologia,* Vol. LXVII, No. 4 (1975).

22. *Mycologia,* Vo. LXIX, No. 4 (1977).

23. Robert Cathcart, MD, "Vitamin C titrating to bowel tolerance," *Medical Hypothesis,* Vol. 7 (1981), pp. 1359-76.

24. *American Journal of Clinical Nutrition,* Vol. 37, No. 5 (1983), pp. 786.

25. *Dermatologia,* No. 156 (1978), pp. 257-67.

26. Brown and Binkley, *Yeast: A Brief Description of Common Sources* (1980).

27. Personal communication to author, 1983.

28. Robert Forman, PhD, *How to Control Your Allergies* (Larchmont Books, 1979.)

29. John Ott, *Light Radiation and You* (Devin Adair, 1982).

30. Kenneth Cooper, *The New Aerobics* (Bantam, 1977).

31. Leon Chaitow, *Your Complete Stress-Proofing Program* (Thorsons, 1984).

32. Editorial, *New England Journal of Medicine,* Dec. 10, 1981; Editorial, *Lancet,* Dec. 12, 1981.

33. Dr. J. Sorenson, "Therapeutic and medicinal uses of copper

aspirinate," in *Copper: Its Medicinal and Biological Effects* (Academic Press, 1979).

34. Personal communication to author, 1984.

35. *Journal of Orthomolecular Psychiatry,* Vol. 13, No. 2 (1984), pp. 66-93.

36. Betsy Russel Manning, "How Safe are Mercury Fillings?," Report to the Cancer Control Society, Los Angeles, 1984.

37. *Health Consciousness,* April 1984, pp. 18-24.

38. *Holistic Medicine* (USA), June-July 1984, p. 29.

39. Robert A. Da Prato, MD, "Fatty Acid Ion Exchange Complexes in Treatment of Candida Albicans." Report by Arteria Co., Concord, California.

40. I. Neuhauser, *Arch. Int. Med.,* Vol. 93, pp. 53-60.

INDEX